Alcohol Information for Teens

Second Edition

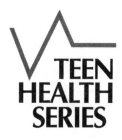

TEEN HEALTH SERIES

Second Edition

Alcohol Information for Teens

Health Tips about Alcohol and Alcoholism

Including Facts about Alcohol's Effects on the Body, Brain, and Behavior, the Consequences of Underage Drinking, Alcohol Abuse Prevention and Treatment, and Coping with Alcoholic Parents

◆

Edited by Lisa Bakewell

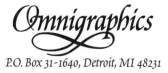

Omnigraphics

P.O. Box 31-1640, Detroit, MI 48231

Bibliographic Note
Because this page cannot legibly accommodate all the copyright notices, the Bibliographic Note portion of the Preface constitutes an extension of the copyright notice.

Edited by Lisa Bakewell

Teen Health Series

Karen Bellenir, *Managing Editor*
David A. Cooke, M.D., *Medical Consultant*
Elizabeth Collins, *Research and Permissions Coordinator*
Cherry Edwards, *Permissions Assistant*
EdIndex, Services for Publishers, *Indexers*

* * *

Omnigraphics, Inc.
Matthew P. Barbour, *Senior Vice President*
Kevin M. Hayes, *Operations Manager*

* * *

Peter E. Ruffner, *Publisher*

Copyright © 2009 Omnigraphics, Inc.
ISBN 978-0-7808-1043-3

Library of Congress Cataloging-in-Publication Data

Alcohol information for teens : health tips about alcohol and alcoholism
including facts about alcohol's effects on the body, brain, and behavior,
the consequences of underage drinking, alcohol abuse prevention and
treatment, and coping with alcoholic parents / edited by Lisa Bakewell.
   p. cm.
   Summary: "Provides basic consumer health information for teens on the
health effects of alcohol use, along with facts about identifying alcohol
problems, and prevention and treatment strategies. Includes index, resource
information and recommendations for further reading"--Provided by publisher.
   Includes bibliographical references and index.
   ISBN 978-0-7808-1043-3 (hardcover : alk. paper) 1.
Alcohol--Physiological effect. 2. Alcoholism--Prevention. 3.
Youth--Alcohol use. I. Bakewell, Lisa.
   QP801.A3A4275 2009
   613.81--dc22

                                                                2009014072

Table Of Contents

Part Three: Alcohol's Effect On Mental Health And Behavior

Part Four: Alcohol Abuse And Alcoholism

Part Five: Preventing Teen Alcohol Use

Part Six: Children Of Alcoholics

Part Seven: If You Need More Information

viii

Preface

About This Book

Underage drinking can lead to a host of negative consequences, including trouble in relationships, in school, and in social activities. Alcohol is also a leading contributor to fatal injuries, and it plays a roll in risky sexual behaviors. Furthermore, alcohol affects every organ in the body, and excessive consumption is associated with multiple adverse health consequences, including liver disease, various cancers, cardiovascular disease, neurological damage, and mental health disorders. In fact, the Centers for Disease Control and Prevention claims that excessive alcohol consumption is the third leading preventable cause of death in the United States, associated with 75,000 deaths per year.

Alcohol Information for Teens, Second Edition provides updated information about alcohol and its effects on the body, brain, and behavior, including short-term consequences and long-term health risks to individual organs and mental well-being. It describes the risks and signs of emerging alcohol-related problems, offers information about treatments, and describes strategies to prevent teen alcohol abuse. A special section offers facts and encouragement to children of alcoholics, and the book concludes with directories of resources for further help and information.

How To Use This Book

This book is divided into parts and chapters. Parts focus on broad areas of interest; chapters are devoted to single topics within a part.

Part One: Basic Information About Alcohol provides a brief introduction to the cultural uses of alcohol, the different categories of alcoholic beverages, and the fermentation process. It discusses why some people choose to drink and why others choose to abstain. The part also summarizes statistical data about underage drinking and describes the consequences associated with it.

Part Two: Alcohol's Effect On The Body discusses the short-term physical consequences of alcohol use, including impaired coordination, diminished reflexes, and the increased risk of death and injury from burns, falls, drowning, alcohol poisoning, and suicide. It also describes the longer-term health consequences associated with heavy drinking and its impact on the brain, heart, stomach, liver, and other body organs.

Part Three: Alcohol's Effect On Mental Health And Behavior explains how alcohol interferes with the ability to form new, long-term memories, and it describes the factors that contribute to alcohol-induced blackouts. It also discusses mental health concerns associated with alcohol use, and it outlines the ways in which alcohol can affect judgment, making drinkers more likely to participate in risky behaviors, including aggression, recklessness, sexual risk taking, and driving while intoxicated.

Part Four: Alcohol Abuse And Alcoholism explains the risk factors for alcoholism and its associated symptoms, including craving, loss of control, physical dependence, and tolerance. It describes the tools medical professionals use in diagnosing alcoholism, the process of seeking help, issues associated with alcohol withdrawal, and the types of treatment most commonly used in the recovery process.

Part Five: Preventing Teen Alcohol Use identifies common tracks of alcohol use and abuse through adolescence and young adulthood. It discusses various ways teens can avoid alcohol-related problems or help friends who may have problems. It also describes how communities can intervene, and it includes facts about the minimum legal drinking age and efforts to deter alcohol-impaired driving, including sobriety checkpoints, alcohol sensors, and zero tolerance laws.

Part Six: Children Of Alcoholics addresses the special concerns of children and teens who are exposed to a parent's alcohol use disorder, including how alcohol abuse disrupts family functioning, how genetic and environmental factors may place children of alcoholics at risk for developing alcohol-related problems, and how teens can cope with parents who are problem drinkers. The part concludes with information about programs designed to help teens escape from a multigenerational cycle of alcoholism.

Part Seven: If You Need More Information includes a list of material for additional reading, a directory of support groups for alcoholics and children of alcoholics, a directory of national resources for additional information about alcohol and alcoholism, and a directory of state agencies for alcohol-treatment referrals.

Bibliographic Note

This volume contains documents and excerpts from publications issued by the following government agencies: Centers for Disease Control and Prevention; Federal Trade Commission; National Cancer Institute; National Clearinghouse for Alcohol and Drug Information; National Digestive Diseases Information Clearinghouse; National Heart, Lung, and Blood Institute; National Highway Traffic Safety Administration; National Institute of Arthritis and Musculoskeletal and Skin Diseases; National Institute of Diabetes and Digestive and Kidney Diseases; National Institute on Alcohol Abuse and Alcoholism; Office of National Drug Control Policy; Office of the Surgeon General; Office on Women's Health; Substance Abuse and Mental Health Services Administration; Surveillance, Epidemiology and End Results (SEER) Program; U.S. Department of Agriculture; U.S. Department of Health and Human Services; and the U.S. Department of Justice.

In addition, this volume contains copyrighted documents and articles produced by the following organizations: A.D.A.M., Inc.; American Academy of Family Physicians; Do It Now Foundation; Insurance Institute for Highway Safety, Highway Loss Data Institute; National Alliance of Advocates for Buprenorphine Treatment; National Association for Children of Alcoholics; National Council on Alcoholism and Drug Dependence; Nemours Foundation; PBS - It's My Life (pbskids.org/itsmylife); University of Notre Dame, Office of Alcohol and Drug Education; and West Virginia University, Community Health Promotion.

Full citation information is provided on the first page of each chapter. Every effort has been made to secure all necessary rights to reprint the copyrighted material. If any omissions have been made, please contact Omnigraphics to make corrections for future editions.

Acknowledgements

In addition to the organizations who have contributed to this book, special thanks are due to research and permissions coordinator, Liz Collins; permissions assistant, Cherry Edwards; editorial assistant, Nicole Salerno; and prepress technician, Elizabeth Bellenir.

About The *Teen Health Series*

At the request of librarians serving today's young adults, the *Teen Health Series* was developed as a specially focused set of volumes within Omnigraphics' *Health Reference Series*. Each volume deals comprehensively with a topic selected according to the needs and interests of people in middle school and high school.

Teens seeking preventive guidance, information about disease warning signs, medical statistics, and risk factors for health problems will find answers to their questions in the *Teen Health Series*. The *Series*, however, is not intended to serve as a tool for diagnosing illness, in prescribing treatments, or as a substitute for the physician/patient relationship. All people concerned about medical symptoms or the possibility of disease are encouraged to seek professional care from an appropriate health care provider.

If there is a topic you would like to see addressed in a future volume of the *Teen Health Series*, please write to:

Editor

Teen Health Series

Omnigraphics, Inc.

P.O. Box 31-1640

Detroit, MI 48231

A Note About Spelling And Style

Teen Health Series editors use *Stedman's Medical Dictionary* as an authority for questions related to the spelling of medical terms and the *Chicago Manual of Style* for questions related to grammatical structures, punctuation, and other editorial concerns. Consistent adherence is not always possible, however, because the individual volumes within the *Series* include many documents from a wide variety of different producers and copyright holders, and the editor's primary goal is to present material from each source as accurately as is possible following the terms specified by each document's producer. This sometimes means that information in different chapters or sections may follow other guidelines and alternate spelling authorities. For example, occasionally a copyright holder may require that eponymous terms be shown in possessive forms (Crohn's disease vs. Crohn disease) or that British spelling norms be retained (leukaemia vs. leukemia).

Locating Information Within The *Teen Health Series*

The *Teen Health Series* contains a wealth of information about a wide variety of medical topics. As the *Series* continues to grow in size and scope, locating the precise information needed by a specific student may become more challenging. To address this concern, information about books within the *Teen Health Series* is included in *A Contents Guide to the Health Reference Series*. The *Contents Guide* presents an extensive list of more than 15,000 diseases, treatments, and other topics of general interest compiled from the Tables of Contents and major index headings from the books of the *Teen Health Series* and *Health Reference Series*. To access *A Contents Guide to the Health Reference Series*, visit www.healthreferenceseries.com.

Our Advisory Board

We would like to thank the following advisory board members for providing guidance to the development of this *Series*:

Dr. Lynda Baker, Associate Professor of Library and Information Science, Wayne State University, Detroit, MI

Nancy Bulgarelli, William Beaumont Hospital Library, Royal Oak, MI

xiv

Karen Imarisio, Bloomfield Township Public Library,
Bloomfield Township, MI

Karen Morgan, Mardigian Library,
University of Michigan-Dearborn, Dearborn, MI

Rosemary Orlando, St. Clair Shores Public Library,
St. Clair Shores, MI

Medical Consultant

Medical consultation services are provided to the *Teen Health Series* editors by David A. Cooke, M.D. Dr. Cooke is a graduate of Brandeis University, and he received his M.D. degree from the University of Michigan. He completed residency training at the University of Wisconsin Hospital and Clinics. He is board-certified in internal medicine. Dr. Cooke currently works as part of the University of Michigan Health System and practices in Ann Arbor, MI. In his free time, he enjoys writing, science fiction, and spending time with his family.

Part One

Basic Information About Alcohol

Chapter 1

What Is Alcohol?

Alcohol has a long history. It has been used in religious ceremonies, as a medicine, and socially for thousands of years. Laws and codes of conduct governing its use and misuse have been a part of human culture throughout history. Some people can use alcohol occasionally and responsibly, while for others the effect of alcohol can be devastating. Herein lies the complexity of alcohol use.

Alcohol is a psychoactive substance, which means that it has the ability to change consciousness and to alter perceptions and behavior. The alcohol found in beverages is known as ethanol or ethyl alcohol. This is the only type of alcohol that is safe to consume, and then only in small quantities.

While there is much controversy over the many problems associated with alcohol, the fact is that a large segment of the population chooses to consume alcoholic beverages. Many people begin drinking during early adolescence. The use of alcohol by college students is a major problem. People in their 20s and 30s comprise the group most often arrested for drunkenness and for driving while intoxicated. However, even senior citizens are not immune to alcohol abuse.

About This Chapter: This chapter includes information from "What Is Alcohol?" "Production of Alcohol," and "Types of Alcoholic Beverages," © 1999-2000 West Virginia University Community Health Promotion. Reprinted with permission. Despite the older dates of these publications, the information they contain is still useful for understanding the history, production, and use of alcoholic beverages.

♣ **It's A Fact!!**

It is difficult for many people to ascertain exactly how much alcohol is found in a drink. A good rule of thumb is that a 12-ounce, 10 proof beer is equal to a five-ounce glass of 24 proof wine, which is equal to a 1½ ounce shot (jigger) of 80 proof hard liquor (distilled spirits). Each of these drinks contains 0.6 ounces of alcohol. To determine how much ethanol (alcohol) is in a drink, divide the proof by half, and then divide that number by 100. Multiply the result by the number of ounces in the drink. Remember that proof is twice the percent of alcohol.

Source: From "Types of Alcoholic Beverages," © 1999-2000 West Virginia University Community Health Promotion. Reprinted with permission.

Approximately half of all alcohol is consumed by just ten percent of the drinking population. A host of social issues plagues this group of heavy drinkers. Lost work time, family pathologies, and medical factors are just a few of the complications associated with alcohol abuse.

Production Of Alcohol

Fermentation is a natural process in which airborne yeast settles on over-ripe fruits, honey, grain products, etc. and feeds on the sugars. The yeast breaks down certain starches in the sugars, and from this process ethyl alcohol and carbon dioxide are produced. In natural fermentation, when the alcohol content reaches a potency of approximately 14 to 15 percent, the process ends.

Distillation of alcohol increases its potency. This process, which was first developed around 800 AD, involves collecting the steam from boiled alcoholic mash (wine, fruit, grain, etc.). The steam, which has a higher alcoholic content, is collected in a special apparatus. When cooled, the resulting liquid has a high alcohol content and a low water volume.

The term proof is a measurement of the alcohol content of a beverage. Proof can be defined as twice the alcohol content of a drink. For example, a bottle of liquor that is designated as 110 proof would contain 55 percent alcohol.

Types Of Alcoholic Beverages

The alcoholic content in a beverage is determined relative to its proof, which is twice the alcohol content. For example, a glass of 24 proof wine would be 12 percent alcohol. A drink that is 40 percent alcohol would be 80 proof. There are three main categories of alcoholic drinks: beer, wine, and distilled spirits (hard liquor).

Beer making has a long history. As far back as 2000 BC, the Code of Hammurabi set standards for beer production and behavioral codes pertaining to drunkenness. Beer is made from grain, malt, hops, yeast, and water. Historically, beer was full-bodied and quite nutritious. The beer of today is highly filtered and of negligible nutritious value, although calorie-laden. The alcohol content of beer in the United States is generally between three and six percent. Grain drinks with a higher level of alcohol are called malts, lager, or ale.

Wine also has a long history. Historically, many monasteries have been known for their wine production. A number of fruits can be used to make wine, including grapes, berries, or peaches. The fruits are crushed, and yeast may be added. In general, the darker the color of wine, the longer the aging process. American wine is approximately nine to 14 percent alcohol. Fortified wines are those with an alcohol content higher than 14 percent. Such wines contain added alcohol or brandy to increase the alcohol content to approximately 20 percent.

The remaining major category of alcoholic drink is distilled spirits, often called "hard liquor." The natural fermentation process stops when the alcohol content reaches 14 percent. However, the discovery of the distillation process by the Arabs led to the use of this type of beverage with its higher alcoholic content. Distillation involves heating the substance of choice and capturing the steam that is released. When cooled, the steam contains less water and more alcohol. A number of different products are used for distilled spirits including corn (bourbon), potatoes (vodka), sugar cane (rum), wine (brandy), and malts/grains (scotch).

♣ It's A Fact!!

Other types of alcohol are not safe to drink. They can be toxic and even fatal if consumed. They include:

- **Butyl Alcohol:** Or butanol. This type of alcohol, derived from butane, is commonly used in products such as adhesives and varnishes.

- **Methyl Alcohol:** Also known as methanol or wood alcohol. It is used in the manufacture of formaldehyde and as industrial solvent. During Prohibition wood alcohol gained notoriety as a mixing agent with ethyl alcohol to make liquor. Several people became blind after drinking this toxic mixture, as methyl alcohol causes swelling of the optic nerve, an irreversible condition.

- **Isopropyl Alcohol:** Also known as rubbing alcohol, is a common household product. It is used as a disinfectant and as an ingredient in cologne and after-shave lotion.

- **Ethylene Glycol:** Also known as antifreeze, is the most harmful type of alcohol. It should never be consumed, as it is deadly.

Source: From "Types of Alcoholic Beverages," © 1999-2000 West Virginia University Community Health Promotion. Reprinted with permission.

Chapter 2

Alcohol Myths And Facts

Underage Drinking: Myths Vs. Facts

You probably see and hear a lot about alcohol—from TV, movies, music, and your friends. But what are the real facts about underage alcohol use? Here are some common myths—and sobering facts—about alcohol use:

MYTH: **Alcohol isn't as harmful as other drugs.** Alcohol increases your risk for many deadly diseases such as cancer. Drinking too much alcohol too quickly can lead to alcohol poisoning, which can kill you.

MYTH: **Drinking is a good way to loosen up at parties.** Drinking is a dumb way to loosen up. It can make you act silly, say things you shouldn't say, and do things you wouldn't normally do (like get into fights or have sex).

MYTH: **Drinking alcohol will make me cool.** There's nothing cool about stumbling around, passing out, or puking on yourself. Drinking alcohol also can cause bad breath and weight gain.

MYTH: **All of the other kids drink alcohol. I need to drink to fit in.** If you really want to fit in, stay sober. Most young people don't drink alcohol.

About This Chapter: This chapter includes information from "Underage Drinking: Myths Vs. Facts," Substance Abuse and Mental Health Services Administration (SAMHSA), 2007; and excerpts from "Tips For Teens: The Truth About Alcohol," SAMHSA, 2006.

Research shows that more than 70 percent of youth aged 12 to 20 haven't had a drink in the past month.

MYTH: **I can sober up quickly by taking a cold shower or drinking coffee.** On average, it takes two to three hours for a single drink to leave the body. Nothing can speed up the process, including drinking coffee, taking a cold shower, or "walking it off."

♣ **It's A Fact!!**

Alcohol Myths

I can drink and still be in control. Drinking impairs your judgement, which increases the likelihood that you will do something you'll later regret such as having unprotected sex, being involved in date rape, damaging property, or being victimized by others.

Drinking isn't all that dangerous. One in three 18 to 24-year-olds are admitted to emergency rooms for serious injuries is intoxicated. And alcohol is also associated with homicides, suicides, and drownings.

It's okay for me to drink to keep up with my boyfriend. Women process alcohol differently. No matter how much he drinks, if you drink the same amount as your boyfriend, you will be more intoxicated and more impaired.

I can manage to drive well enough after a few drinks. About one-half of all fatal traffic crashes among 18 to 24-year-olds involve alcohol. If you are under 21, driving after drinking any alcohol is illegal and you could lose your license. The risk of a fatal crash for drivers with a positive blood alcohol content (BAC), compared with other drivers, increases with increasing BAC. The risks also increase more steeply for drivers younger than age 21 than for older drivers.

I'd be better off if I learn to "hold my liquor." If you have to drink increasingly larger amounts of alcohol to get a "buzz" or get "high," you are developing tolerance. Tolerance is actually a warning sign that you're developing more serious problems with alcohol.

Source: "Alcohol Myths," National Institute on Alcohol Abuse and Alcoholism (NIAAA), July 2007.

MYTH: **Adults drink, so kids should be able to drink too.** A young person's brain and body are still growing. Drinking alcohol can cause learning problems or lead to adult alcoholism. People who begin drinking by age 15 are five times more likely to abuse or become dependent on alcohol than those who begin drinking after age 20.

MYTH: **Beer and wine are safer than liquor.** Alcohol is alcohol...it can cause you problems no matter how you consume it. One 12-ounce bottle of beer or a 5-ounce glass of wine (about a half-cup) has as much alcohol as a 1.5-ounce shot of liquor. Alcopops—sweet drinks laced with malt liquor—often contain more alcohol than beer.

MYTH: **I can drink alcohol and not have any problems.** If you're under 21, drinking alcohol is a big problem. It's illegal. If caught, you may have to pay a fine, perform community service, or take alcohol awareness classes. Kids who drink are also more likely to get poor grades in school and are at a higher risk for being a crime victim.

Tips For Teens: The Truth About Alcohol

Get The Facts

FACT: **Alcohol affects your brain.** Drinking can lead to a loss of coordination, poor judgment, slowed reflexes, distorted vision, memory lapses, and even blackouts.

FACT: **Alcohol affects your body.** Alcohol can damage every organ in your body. It is absorbed directly into your bloodstream and can increase your risk for a variety of life-threatening diseases, including cancer.

FACT: **Alcohol affects your self-control.** Alcohol can depress your central nervous system, lower your inhibitions, and impair your judgment. Drinking can lead to risky behaviors, such as driving when you shouldn't or having unprotected sex.

FACT: **Alcohol can kill you.** Drinking large amounts of alcohol at one time—or very rapidly—can cause alcohol poisoning, which can lead to coma or even death. Driving and drinking also can be deadly. In 2003, thirty-one

♣ It's A Fact!!
Know The Signs

How can you tell if a friend has a drinking problem? Sometimes it's tough to tell. But there are signs you can look for. If your friend has one or more of the following warning signs, he or she may have a problem with alcohol.

• Getting drunk on a regular basis

• Lying about how much alcohol he or she is using

• Believing that alcohol is necessary to have fun

• Having frequent hangovers

• Feeling run-down, depressed, or even suicidal

• Having "blackouts" (forgetting what he or she did while drinking)

What can you do to help someone who has a drinking problem? Be a real friend. You might even save a life. Encourage your friend to stop or seek professional help. For information and referrals, call the National Clearinghouse for Alcohol and Drug Information at 800-729-6686.

Source: Excerpted from "Tips For Teens: The Truth About Alcohol," Substance Abuse and Mental Health Services Administration (SAMHSA), 2006.

percent of drivers age 15 to 20 who died in traffic accidents had been drinking alcohol.

FACT: Alcohol can hurt you—even if you're not the one drinking. If you're around people who are drinking, you have an increased risk of being seriously injured, involved in car crashes, or affected by violence. At the very least, you may have to deal with people who are sick, out of control, or unable to take care of themselves.

Before You Risk It

Know The Law. It is illegal to buy or possess alcohol if you are under age 21.

Get The Facts. One drink can make you fail a breath test. In some states, people under age 21 can lose their driver's license, be subject to a heavy fine, or have their car permanently taken away.

Stay Informed. "Binge" drinking means having five or more drinks on one occasion. Studies show that more than 35 percent of adults, with an alcohol problem, developed symptoms—such as binge drinking—by age 19.

Know The Risks. Alcohol is a drug. Mixing it with any other drug can be extremely dangerous. Alcohol and acetaminophen—a common ingredient in over-the-counter (OTC) pain and fever reducers—can damage your liver. Alcohol mixed with other drugs can cause nausea, vomiting, fainting, heart problems, and difficulty breathing. Mixing alcohol and drugs also can lead to coma and death.

Keep Your Edge. Alcohol is a depressant—or downer—because it reduces brain activity. If you are depressed before you start drinking, alcohol can make you feel worse.

Look Around You. Most teens aren't drinking alcohol. Research shows that 71 percent of people 12–20 haven't had a drink in the past month.

Chapter 3

Frequently Asked Questions About Alcohol

Introduction To Alcohol

What is alcohol?

Ethyl alcohol (or ethanol) is an intoxicating ingredient found in beer, wine, and liquor. Alcohol is produced by the fermentation of yeast, sugars, and starches.

How does alcohol affect a person?

Alcohol affects every organ in the body. It is a central nervous system depressant that is rapidly absorbed from the stomach and small intestine into the bloodstream. Alcohol is metabolized in the liver by enzymes, however the liver can only metabolize a small amount of alcohol at a time, so the excess alcohol circulates throughout the body. The intensity of the effect of alcohol on the body is directly related to the amount consumed.

Why do some people react differently to alcohol than others?

Individual reactions to alcohol vary and are influenced by many factors. Factors that could influence individual reactions to alcohol are listed below.

About This Chapter: This chapter includes information from "Alcohol: Frequently Asked Questions," Centers for Disease Control and Prevention (CDC), reviewed April 2, 2008.

- Age

- Gender

- Race or ethnicity

- Physical condition (weight, fitness level, etc.)

- Amount of food consumed before drinking

- How quickly the alcohol was consumed

- Use of drugs or prescription medicines

- Family history of alcohol problems

> **♣ It's A Fact!!**
>
> A standard drink is equal to 13.7 grams (0.6 ounces) of pure alcohol. Since alcohol-containing drinks aren't made of pure alcohol, a standard drink may vary in size depending on the type of alcohol.
>
> - 12 ounces of beer
>
> - Eight ounces of malt liquor
>
> - Five ounces of wine
>
> - A "shot" (1.5 ounces) of 80-proof distilled spirits or liquor such as gin, rum, vodka, and whiskey

Is beer or wine safer to drink than hard liquor?

No. One 12-ounce beer has about the same amount of alcohol as one 5-ounce glass of wine or 1.5-ounce shot of liquor. It is the amount of ethanol consumed that affects a person most, not the type of alcoholic drink.

Drinking Levels

What does moderate drinking mean?

There is no one definition of moderate drinking, but generally the term is used to describe low-risk or responsible drinking. According to the Dietary Guidelines for Americans, drinking in moderation is defined as having no more than one drink per day for women and no more than two drinks per day for men. This definition refers to the amount consumed on any single day and is not intended as an average over several days.

Is it safe to drink alcohol and drive?

No. Alcohol use slows reaction time and impairs judgment and coordination—all skills needed to drive a car safely. The more alcohol consumed, the greater the impairment.

What does it mean to be above the legal limit for drinking?

The legal limit for drinking is the alcohol level above which an individual is subject to legal penalties such as arrest or loss of driver's license.

- Legal limits are measured using either a blood alcohol test or a breathalyzer test.

- Legal limits are typically defined by state law and may vary based on individual characteristics such as age and occupation.

♣ It's A Fact!!

Legal limits do not define a level below which it is safe to operate a vehicle or engage in some other activity. Impairment due to alcohol use begins to occur at levels well below the legal limit.

All states in the United States have adopted 0.08% (80 mg/dL) as the legal limit for operating a motor vehicle for drivers aged 21 years or older. However, drivers under the age of 21 are not allowed to operate a motor vehicle with any level of alcohol in their system.

How do I know if it's okay to drink?

The current Dietary Guidelines for Americans recommend that if adults choose to drink alcoholic beverages, they do not exceed one drink per day for women and two drinks per day for men. These guidelines also specify that there are some people who should not drink alcoholic beverages all, such as those listed below.

- Children and adolescents

- Individuals of any age who cannot restrict their drinking to moderate levels

- Women who may become pregnant or who are pregnant

- Individuals who plan to drive, operate machinery, or take part in other activities that requires attention, skill, or coordination

- Individuals taking prescription or over-the-counter medications that can interact with alcohol

- Individuals with specific medical conditions
- Persons recovering from alcoholism

Excessive Alcohol Use

What is meant by heavy drinking?

For men, heavy drinking is typically defined as consuming an average of more than two drinks per day. For women, heavy drinking is typically defined as consuming an average of more than one drink per day.

What is binge drinking?

According to the National Institute on Alcohol Abuse and Alcoholism, binge drinking is defined as a pattern of alcohol consumption that brings the blood alcohol concentration (BAC) level to 0.08% or above. This pattern of drinking usually corresponds to five or more drinks on a single occasion for men or four or more drinks on a single occasion for women, generally within about two hours.

What is the difference between alcoholism and alcohol abuse?

Alcoholism (or alcohol dependence) is a diagnosable disease characterized by several factors including a strong craving for alcohol, continued use despite harm or personal injury, the inability to limit drinking, physical illness when drinking stops, and the need to increase the amount drunk in order to feel the effects.

Alcohol abuse is a pattern of drinking that results in harm to one's health, interpersonal relationships, or ability to work. Certain manifestations of alcohol abuse include failure to fulfill responsibilities at work, school, or home; drinking in dangerous situations such as while driving; legal problems associated with alcohol use; and continued drinking despite problems caused or worsened by drinking. Alcohol abuse can lead to alcohol dependence.

What does it mean to get drunk?

"Getting drunk" or intoxicated is the result of consuming excessive amounts of alcohol. Binge drinking typically results in acute intoxication.

♣ **It's A Fact!!**

Alcohol intoxication can be detrimental to health for a variety of reasons, including—but not limited to—those listed here:

- Impaired brain function resulting in poor judgment, reduced reaction time, loss of balance and motor skills, and/or slurred speech

- Dilation of blood vessels causing a feeling of warmth, but resulting in rapid loss of body heat

- Increased risk of certain cancers, stroke, and liver diseases (such as cirrhosis) particularly when excessive amounts of alcohol are consumed over extended periods of time

- Damage to a developing fetus if consumed by pregnant women

- Increased risk of motor-vehicle traffic crashes, violence, and other injuries

Also, coma and death can occur if alcohol is consumed rapidly and in large amounts due to depression of the central nervous system

Drinking Problems

How do I know if I have a drinking problem?

Drinking is a problem if it causes trouble in your relationships, in school, in social activities, or in how you think and feel. If you are concerned that either you or someone in your family might have a drinking problem, consult your personal physician.

What can I do if I or someone I know has a drinking problem?

Consult your personal physician if you feel that you or someone you know has a drinking problem. Another resource, the National Drug and Alcohol Treatment Referral Routing Service, is available at 1-800-662-HELP. This service can provide you with information about treatment programs in your local community and allow you to speak with someone about alcohol problems.

What health problems are associated with excessive alcohol use?

Excessive drinking—both in the form of heavy drinking or binge drinking—is associated with numerous health problems and injury, including (but not limited to) those listed here:

- Chronic diseases such as liver cirrhosis (damage to liver cells), pancreatitis (inflammation of the pancreas), and various cancers including liver, mouth, throat, larynx (the voice box), and esophagus

- High blood pressure and psychological disorders

- Unintentional injuries such as motor-vehicle traffic crashes, falls, drowning, burns, and firearm injuries

- Violence such as child maltreatment, homicide, and suicide

- Harm to a developing fetus if a woman drinks while pregnant

- Alcohol abuse or dependence

Special Populations

I'm young. Is drinking bad for my health?

Yes. Studies have shown that alcohol use by youth and young adults increases the risk of both fatal and nonfatal injuries. Research has also shown that youth who use alcohol before age 15 are five times more likely to become alcohol dependent than adults who begin at age 21. Other consequences of youth alcohol use include increased risky sexual behaviors, poor school performance, and risk of suicide and homicide.

Is it okay to drink when pregnant?

No. There is no safe level of alcohol use during pregnancy. Women who are pregnant or plan on becoming pregnant should refrain from drinking alcohol. Several conditions, including fetal alcohol syndrome disorders have been linked to alcohol use during pregnancy. Women of childbearing age should also avoid binge drinking to reduce the risk of unintended pregnancy and potential exposure of a developing fetus to alcohol.

Chapter 4

Understanding Why Young Adults Drink Alcohol

Too often today's headlines bring news of yet another alcohol-related tragedy involving a young person—a case of fatal alcohol poisoning on a college campus or a late-night drinking and driving crash—but are they really at higher risk than anyone else for problems involving alcohol?

Some of the most important new data to emerge on young adult drinking was collected through a nationwide survey, the National Epidemiologic Survey on Alcohol and Related Conditions (NESARC). According to the data, in 2001–2002 about 70 percent of young adults in the United States, or about 19 million people, consumed alcohol in the year preceding the survey.

It's not only that young people are drinking, but it's the way they drink that puts them at such high risk for alcohol-related problems. Research consistently shows that people tend to drink the heaviest in their late teens and early to mid-twenties. Young adults are especially likely to binge drink and to drink heavily. According to NESARC data, about 46 percent of young adults (12.4 million) engaged in drinking that exceeded the recommended daily limits at least once in the past year, and 14.5 percent of young adults

About This Chapter: This chapter includes excerpts from "Alcohol Alert: Young Adult Drinking," National Institute on Alcohol Abuse and Alcoholism (NIAAA), April 2006. The complete text of this document, including references can be found online at http://pubs.niaaa.nih.gov/publications/aa68/aa68.htm.

♣ It's A Fact!!

It is possible to drink legally and safely—when a person is 21 or older and drinks in fairly small amounts. But if you're under 21—or if you drink too much at any age—alcohol can be especially risky. A few of the dangers of underage drinking include death, addiction, thinking problems, and arrest.

Drinking too soon or too much can affect your mood and your thinking; can hurt others, get you in legal trouble, and damage your relationships; can harm your body now and when you grow up; and can get you hooked.

Source: "Too Much, Too Soon, Too Risky," National Institute on Alcohol Abuse and Alcoholism (http://www.thecoolspot.gov) 2004.

(3.9 million) had an average consumption that exceeded the recommended weekly limits.

Such risky drinking often leads to tragic consequences—most notably alcohol-related traffic fatalities. Thirty-two percent of drivers ages 16–20 who died in traffic crashes in 2003 had measurable alcohol in their blood, and 51 percent of drivers ages 21–24 who died tested positive for alcohol. Clearly, young adult drinkers pose a serious public health threat, putting themselves and others at risk.

An Age Of Exploration

Young adulthood is a stage of life marked by change and exploration. People move out of their parents' homes and into dormitories or houses with peers. They go to college, begin to work full-time, and form serious relationships. They explore their own identities and how they fit in the world. The roles of parents weaken and the influences of peers gain greater strength. Young adults are on their own for the first time, free to make their own decisions, including the decision to drink alcohol.

Young adulthood also is the time during which young people obtain the education and training they need for future careers. Mastery of these endeavors is vital to future success. Problems with school and work can produce frustration and stress, which can lead to a variety of unhealthy behaviors—including increased drinking. Conversely, alcohol use during this important time of transition can impede the successful mastery of these developmental tasks, also increasing stress.

Factors That Influence Use

Outside influences as well as individual characteristics help determine whether a person will begin drinking and how much he or she will consume.

- **Gender:** Men are much more likely than women to drink in ways that are harmful. As shown in a recent national survey of 19- to 30-year-olds, 45 percent of men and 26.7 percent of women reported heavy drinking in the past two weeks, and 7.4 percent of men and three percent of women reported daily drinking.

- **Race And Ethnicity:** Racial, ethnic, and cultural differences in drinking and alcohol-related problems also have been documented. In general, white and Native American young adults drink more than African Americans and Asians, and drinking rates for Hispanics fall in the middle.

- **Peer Influences:** People entering college or the workforce may be especially vulnerable to the influence of peers because of their need to make new friendships. And they may increase their drinking in order to gain acceptance by peers.

- **Personality Characteristics:** A number of personality traits have been associated with drinking greater amounts of alcohol and drinking more often, including impulsivity, risk-taking,

---

✎ What's It Mean?

The National Epidemiologic Survey on Alcohol and Related Conditions (NESARC) defined "binge drinking" and "drinking heavily" as follows:

- <u>Binge Drinking</u>: Consuming five or more drinks in a row at least once in the past month.

- <u>Drinking Heavily</u>: Consuming five or more drinks in a row on at least five occasions in the past month.

Source: National Institute on Alcohol Abuse and Alcoholism (NIAAA), April 2006.

and sensation-seeking—or the tendency to seek out new and exciting experiences. Sensation-seeking and impulsivity have also been linked to deviant behavior and nonconformity, both of which are predictors of heavy drinking and related problems among youth.

- **Alcohol Expectancies:** Positive alcohol expectancies—or the belief that drinking will lead to positive, pleasurable experiences—play a key role in the drinking behavior of young adults. What a person expects from drinking not only predicts when he or she will begin drinking, but also how much he or she will drink throughout young adulthood. As people age through adolescence and into young adulthood, they increasingly expect benefits from drinking and become less convinced of the risks.

- **Family Influences:** During young adulthood, parents may have less direct influence on their children's drinking behavior, but they still play a major protective role. The example set by parents with their own drinking has been shown to affect their children's drinking throughout their lifetime. Young people model their behavior after their parents' patterns of consumption (including quantity and frequency), situations and contexts of use, attitudes regarding use, and expectancies. The family's structure and aspects of the parent-child relationship (for example, parenting style, attachment and bonding, nurturance, abuse or neglect, conflict, discipline, and monitoring) also have been linked to young people's alcohol use.

- **Genetics:** Alcohol problems seem to "run" in some families. This family

---

♣ It's A Fact!!

- Some people drink alcohol to feel less tense or anxious and more relaxed.

- Heavier drinking can turn good feelings into bad—and bad feelings into worse. Since alcohol affects memory, people sometimes don't remember feeling bad.

- People who drink heavily often wind up doing things they really didn't want to do. They end up in accidents, fights, and other bad situations that harm property, other people, and themselves.

Source: "Too Much, Too Soon, Too Risky," National Institute on Alcohol Abuse and Alcoholism (http://www.thecoolspot.gov) 2004.

♣ **It's A Fact!!**

The phenomenon of perceived social norms—or the belief that "everyone" is drinking and drinking is acceptable—is one of the strongest correlates of drinking among young adults. Many college students think campus attitudes are much more permissive toward drinking than they really are and believe other students drink much more than they actually do.

Source: National Institute on Alcohol Abuse and Alcoholism (NIAAA), April 2006.

connection to alcoholism may be the result of a genetic link and/or may reflect the child's modeling of drinking behavior. Siblings can also influence drinking through modeling and by providing access to alcohol. It's unclear whether children of alcoholics have different drinking patterns and problems in young adulthood than those who do not have a family history of alcoholism. Research does show, however, that people with a family history of alcoholism are less likely than those with no family history to mature out of heavy drinking as they approach young adulthood.

Other personality traits, such as a feeling of invincibility—that are common among young adults—can influence drinking. Many young people simply do not see themselves as vulnerable to any negative consequences that might occur because of drinking, such as having an accident or becoming dependent on alcohol. This optimistic bias makes young adults more likely to take risks and perhaps to drink excessively, although risk-taking may not be a direct cause of drinking. That is, research shows that the decision to drink is influenced more by the perceived benefits of drinking than by the perceived risks.

Negative moods, feelings of depression, and anxiety disorders also may influence alcohol use. Research has suggested that some people drink to relieve feelings of stress and to cope with negative feelings—a good predictor of heavy drinking as well as drinking problems.

♣ **It's A Fact!!**

Change In Expectations About Alcohol Use In Adolescence

Expectations about the effects of drinking alcohol are measurable in children before they begin to drink and can influence how early a child drinks and how much he or she will drink at initiation.

- Research suggests that people who have expectations of more positive experiences from drinking, tend to drink more than others and are at highest risk for excessive drinking.

- Children, in general, shift from a primary emphasis on the negative or adverse effects of drinking alcohol before about age nine to a primary emphasis on the positive and arousing effects of alcohol by about age 13.

- Those at highest risk for excessive drinking show the largest emphasis on alcohol's positive or arousing effects.

Therefore, it is important to be aware of the messages about alcohol use that youth receive and the attitudes that these messages engender in children and adolescents about alcohol and its use.

Source: From *The Surgeon General's Call To Action To Prevent And Reduce Underage Drinking*, Office of the Surgeon General, U.S. Department of Health and Human Services, 2007.

Conclusion

Research consistently shows that people tend to drink the heaviest in their late teens and early to mid-twenties. This high level of alcohol use comes at an age when people are moving away from parental restrictions but before they take on the full responsibilities of adult life. As young people begin to assume more adult roles—full-time employment, marriage, and parenthood—they often reduce their drinking. This reduction in alcohol use may be a result of the limitations that adult roles place on social activities or may reflect a change in young people's attitudes toward drinking.

Research also shows that young adults who drink in ways that are especially harmful—those who fit the diagnostic criteria for alcohol dependence—may have predisposing personality characteristics and other factors that place them at greater risk for problems with alcohol.

Chapter 5

Underage Drinking:
Understanding The Scope Of The Problem

This chapter summarizes research on the epidemiology of youth drinking, including the consequences of youthful drinking; risk and protective factors and drinking trajectories; and information on special populations at particular risk for drinking-related problems.

Epidemiology Of Underage Drinking

Alcohol is the drug of choice among youth. Young people drink too much and at too early an age, thereby creating problems for themselves, for people around them, and for society as a whole. Hence, underage drinking is a leading public health problem in this country.

Prevalence And Age Of Initiation

Nationwide surveys, as well as studies in smaller populations, show that alcohol drinking is widespread among adolescents. For example, 2004 data from Monitoring the Future (MTF), an annual survey of U.S. youth, show that more than three-fourths of 12th graders, nearly two-thirds of 10th graders,

About This Chapter: This chapter includes excerpts from "The Scope of the Problem," *Alcohol Research and Health*, Vol. 28, No. 3, National Institute on Alcohol Abuse and Alcoholism (NIAAA), 2004/2005. The complete text of this document, including references, is available online at http://pubs.niaaa.nih.gov/publications/arh283/111-120.htm.

and more than two in five eighth graders have consumed alcohol at some point in their lives. And when youth drink, they tend to drink heavily. Underage drinkers consume on average four to five drinks per occasion about five times a month. By comparison, adult drinkers, ages 26 and older, consume on average two to three drinks per occasion about nine times a month. A particularly worrisome aspect of underage drinking is the high prevalence of heavy episodic drinking, defined as drinking five or more drinks in a row in the past two weeks. MTF data show that 12 percent of eighth graders, 22 percent of 10th graders, and 28 percent of 12th graders engage in heavy episodic drinking. It should come as no surprise, then, that about three-fifths of 12th graders, two-fifths of 10th graders, and one-fifth of eighth graders say they have been drunk. In fact, the highest prevalence of dependence is seen in people ages 18 to 24.

Studies also indicate that drinking often begins at very young ages. Data from recent surveys show that approximately 10 percent of nine to 10-year-olds have already started drinking, nearly a third of youth begin drinking before age 13, and more than one-fourth of 14-year-olds report drinking within the past year. Other researchers have documented that drinking becomes

☞ Remember!!

Alcohol is the drug of choice among youth, often with devastating consequences.

- Alcohol is a leading contributor to injury death, the main cause of death for people under age 21.

- Drinking early in life also is associated with an increased risk of developing an alcohol use disorder at some time during the life span.

- Data consistently indicate that rates of drinking and alcohol-related problems are highest among White and American Indian or Alaska Native youth, followed by Hispanic youth, African Americans, and Asians.

- Prevalence rates of drinking for boys and girls are similar in the younger age groups. Among older adolescents, however, more boys than girls engage in frequent and heavy drinking, and boys show higher rates of drinking problems.

increasingly common through the teenage years. In addition, a number of studies have documented that the early onset of alcohol use (usually set at age 13 and younger) as well as the escalation of drinking in adolescence are both risk factors for the development of alcohol-related problems in adulthood.

These findings clearly are cause for concern, as are recent data suggesting that the age of first use of alcohol is declining. These data indicate that the average age of first use among young people of all ages was about 16 in 1999, compared with about 17½ in 1965. Looking at underage drinkers only, 12- to 18-year-olds who report drinking report that they began doing so be- tween two and three years earlier, when they were about nine to 15, respec- tively. This is important because, initiating alcohol consumption earlier in adolescence or in childhood is a marker for later problems, including heavier use of alcohol and other drugs during adolescence and meeting criteria for an alcohol dependence diagnosis in adulthood.

Most of what we know about underage drinking derives from studies of youth ages 12 to 21. To address alcohol-related problems as developmental phenomena, we will need to understand more about what happens before age 12 with regard to alcohol consumption, alcohol awareness, and alcohol expect- ancies among children who have started to drink and among those who have not. A recent Medline search found a dearth of studies addressing drinking by younger children, and the few existing studies that turned up in this search were conducted among non-U.S. populations. Two national data sets, how- ever, address alcohol use by children in sixth grade or below (typically age 12 and younger), albeit imperfectly and far from comprehensively. One is the Partnership Attitude Tracking Study (PATS), carried out for the Partnership for a Drug-Free America in 1993, and annually from 1995 through 1999. The other is the collection of PRIDE surveys carried out during the academic years 1997–1998 through 2001–2002. PATS data reveal a tripling of alcohol experi- ence between fourth and sixth grade: 9.8 percent of fourth graders, 16.1 per- cent of fifth graders, and 29.4 percent of sixth graders report trying more than a sip of alcohol. PRIDE data show similar rates of use in this population. Despite methodological problems with these data sets, PATS and PRIDE show that a nontrivial level of alcohol consumption occurs among a significant proportion of the 12-and-under population.

Consequences

Underage drinking can result in a range of adverse short-term and long-term consequences:

- Academic problems

- Social problems

- Physical problems such as hangovers or medical illnesses

- Unwanted, unintended, and unprotected sexual activity

- Physical and sexual assault

- Memory problems

- Increased risk for suicide and homicide

- Alcohol-related car crashes and other unintentional injuries such as burns, falls, and drownings

- Death from alcohol poisoning

- Alterations in brain development that may have consequences reaching far beyond adolescence

> **☞ Remember!!**
>
> The negative consequences of underage drinking include a range of physical, academic, and social problems. Perhaps most frightening, alcohol is the leading contributor to injury death, the main cause of death for people under age 21. However, alcohol also plays a powerful role in risky sexual behavior, including unwanted, unintended, and unprotected sexual activity, and sex with multiple partners. Alcohol is associated with academic failure and drug use. Over the longer term, data have shown that drinking early in life is associated with an increased risk of developing an alcohol use disorder at some time during the life span.

Alcohol is a leading contributor to injury death, the main cause of death for people under age 21. Annually, about 5,000 youth under age 21 die from alcohol-related injuries that involve underage drinking. This includes injuries sustained in motor vehicle crashes (about 1,900), homicides (about 1,600), and suicides (about 300), as well as unintentional injuries not related to motor vehicle crashes. Furthermore, the role of alcohol in both fatalities and injuries may be significantly underreported, in part because in many states, alcohol involvement in an injury relieves insurance providers of liability for medical expenses, so health care providers may not ask victims about, or report, alcohol use.

Numerous cases of alcohol poisoning, the result of the acute toxic effects of alcohol that can range from gastritis to severe gastrointestinal bleeding to respiratory arrest and death, have been reported in the news media. Although many of these tragedies occur on college campuses, especially striking was the report of two 11-year-old boys found dead of alcohol poisoning in a snowy field on the Flathead Indian Reservation in Montana, with blood alcohol concentration (BAC) levels of 0.20 percent and 0.50 percent. Although alcohol poisoning is by no means a major cause of death among youth, reports such as this underscore the tragic influence that hazardous drinking can wield over youth culture.

In the National Longitudinal Alcohol Epidemiologic Survey (NLAES) of people ages 18 and older in the United States, people who reported starting to drink before the age of 15 were four times more likely to also report meeting the criteria for dependence at some point in their lives. This survey also shows that children who drink at age 14 or younger are much more likely during their lifetimes to sustain unintentional injuries, to get into physical fights, and to become involved in motor vehicle crashes after drinking.

> ### ✎ What's It Mean?
>
> Binge Drinking: The National Institute on Alcohol Abuse and Alcoholism defines binge drinking as a pattern of drinking alcohol that brings blood alcohol concentration (BAC) to 0.08 grams percent or above. For the typical adult, this pattern corresponds to consuming five or more drinks (men), or four or more drinks (women), in about two hours.

Similarly, other survey data indicate that the younger children and adolescents are when they start to drink, the more likely they are to engage in behaviors that can harm themselves and others. Those who start to drink before age 13, for example, are nine times more likely to binge drink frequently (five or more drinks on an occasion at least six times per month) as high school students than those who begin drinking later.

Binge drinking is clearly dangerous for the drinker and for society. Compared with nondrinkers, a greater proportion of frequent binge drinkers (nearly one million high school students nationwide) engaged in other risky behavior in the past 30 days, including carrying a gun (22 percent versus three percent), using marijuana (73 percent versus seven percent), using cocaine (26 percent versus zero percent), and having sex with six or more partners (31 percent versus four percent). In addition, these youth were more likely than abstainers to earn grades that are mostly Ds or Fs in school (15 percent versus five percent), be injured in a fight (13 percent versus two percent), or be injured in a suicide attempt (nine percent versus one percent). The extent to which alcohol use per se makes these other outcomes more likely is yet to be determined. However, the longitudinal evidence is very strong that the risk factors predicting earlier alcohol use also are strong predictors of virtually all of these other consequences.

Risk Trajectories And Drinking Trajectories

Not only do youth begin drinking at different ages but their trajectories of risk also vary considerably, even before alcohol use has begun. Recent work following high-risk populations of children from preschool onward has shown major differences in the trajectories of externalizing and internalizing risk from preschool to early adolescence. These varied as a function of initial level of risk in early childhood, the child's age, and the level of familial risk. Particularly for the externalizing trajectory, children who started out at very high levels of individual and familial risk became indistinguishable from those at lower levels during the early school years, but as these youth moved into early adolescence, the differences reemerged and became amplified, with the highest-risk children increasing the greatest amount. Conversely, the externalizing behavior of children at the lowest level of initial risk who were exposed to the lowest level of familial risk changed the least, although even they increased in level of externalizing behavior as they moved into adolescence.

Similarly, the drinking patterns and practices youth adopt as they grow into young adults—their drinking trajectories—also vary considerably once they start to drink. No single trajectory describes the course of alcohol use for all or even most young people. Research findings provide strong evidence for wide developmental variation in drinking patterns in the population. For example, Steinman and Schulenberg (2003) identified six common trajectories

---

❖ It's A Fact!!

National surveys make it clear that alcohol drinking among youth is both widespread and harmful. Surveys provide data not only on the numbers of middle and high school students who drink but also on how they drink. The data show that when youth drink, they drink heavily in comparison with adults, consuming on average four to five drinks per occasion about five times a month, compared with two to three drinks per occasion about nine times a month for adults.

Studies also find that drinking often begins at very young ages; a recent survey found that more than one-fourth of 14-year-olds reported drinking within the last year.

---

among early and middle adolescents: abstinence, rare use, high school onset, early but nonescalating use, early and gradually escalating use, and consistently high use. In another study, Schulenberg and colleagues (1996b) identified six trajectories of heavy drinking among young people ages 18 to 24: chronic heavy drinkers, decreased, increased, fling (that is, low, high, low), rare, and never. In addition, alcohol abuse treatment and other experiences may influence drinking trajectories. Studying the developmental trajectories of drinking behavior and how various risk and protective factors influence those trajectories is critical to understanding the complexity of underage drinking.

Special Populations Of Young People

Children Of Alcoholics

Children of alcoholics (COAs) are between four and 10 times as likely to become alcoholics themselves as children from families that have no adults with alcoholism. COAs are at elevated risk for earlier onset of drinking and earlier progression into drinking problems. Some of the elevated risk is attributable to exposure and socialization effects found in alcoholic households, some to genetically transmitted differences in response to alcohol that make the drinking more pleasurable and/or less aversive, and some is attributable to elevated transmission of risky temperamental and behavioral traits that lead COAs, more than other youth, into increased contact with earlier-drinking and heavier-drinking peers.

♣ **It's A Fact!!**

Although almost all U.S. youth grow up in a culture permeated by alcohol, they are not uniformly at risk
for alcohol consumption or its consequences. Much research has
addressed the risk and protective factors associated with youth drinking. These factors include but are not limited to family history and
genetic vulnerability, social stressors such as poverty and lack
of social support, family characteristics, alcohol availability, temperament, and other individual factors.

From a public health standpoint, according to NLAES data, approximately 9.7 million children age 17 or younger, or 15 percent of the child
population in that age range, were living in households with one or more
adults classified as having an alcohol abuse or dependence diagnosis during
the past year. Approximately 70 percent of these children were biological,
foster, adopted, or stepchildren. That is, 6.8 million children meet the formal definition of COA, although not all are exposed to the same level of risk
for use, problem use, and alcohol use disorder (AUD). Given that these fig-
ures concern past-year exposure to at least one alcoholic adult, from the perspective of socialization risk, they only reflect acute exposure. Other data
from NLAES provide estimates of the number of children living in a household with an adult who had abused or been dependent on alcohol at some
point; the figure is 43 percent of the under-18 population, or somewhat less
than half of all children. Given the size of this group, any approach to risk
identification will be extremely complex.

A second important consideration is that COA status is heavily used as a
proxy for "alcoholism risk" on the one hand and socialization risk on the
other, but the COA designation more precisely is a proxy for multiple causal
inputs, not all of which may be present in the individual case. Thus, being a
COA implies elevated genetic risk, although the alcoholic genetic diatheses
may not have been passed on to a particular child. One may be a COA without being undercontrolled, having an attention deficit hyperactivity disorder

diagnosis, or other problems known to be associated with increased risk of alcohol dependence.

Socialization risk involves exposure, but given the high divorce rates found in this population, evaluating the level of socialization risk is complex, involving both the quantification of the length of the exposure and the identification of the developmental period during which the socialization took place. Vulnerability is greater during some developmental periods than others. In addition, a substantial amount of marital assortment occurs in alcoholic families. When assortment is present, risk exposure is multiplied, and COA effects become a function of genetic risk(s), individual parent risk, and the synergistic risk created by marital interaction.

Third, the potential for indirect socialization effects also is higher in COAs than in other children. Parental psychopathology has been documented as a risk factor for poorer parental monitoring, which in turn leads to a higher probability of involvement with a deviant peer group, including earlier exposure to alcohol and other drugs.

Fourth, COA risk is not simply risk for the development of AUD. Given what is known about the elevated comorbidities found among offspring of alcoholics, this designator also is a marker of elevated risk for behavioral and cognitive deficits. These include attention deficit disorder, behavioral undercontrol/conduct disorder, delinquency, lower IQ, poor school performance, low self-esteem, and other problems. Furthermore, the evidence strongly implicates some of these non-alcohol-specific characteristics as causal to both problem alcohol use and elevated risk for AUD.

These factors implicate the COA population as an important component of the underage drinking population. For the same reasons, however, it is essential to determine which components of that risk composite are the strongest mediators of the underage-drinking outcome.

College Students

College students are a highly visible group of underage drinkers among whom alcohol consumption is commonplace. Indeed, many college students accept alcohol use as a normal part of student life. Studies consistently indicate that about four in five college students drink alcohol; about two in five engage in episodic heavy consumption, often called bingeing (five or more drinks in a row for men and four or more in a row for women; generally asked with respect to the past two weeks or past 30 days, depending on the survey); and about one in five engages in frequent episodic heavy consumption (bingeing three or more times in the past two weeks).

The consequences of drinking among college students include academic problems, social problems, legal problems, involvement in physical and/or sexual assault or risky sex, and even death. An estimated 1,700 college students, between the ages of 18 and 24, die each year from alcohol-related unintentional injuries including motor vehicle crashes. Another 599,000 students are unintentionally injured while under the influence of alcohol, 696,000 are assaulted by other students who have been drinking, and 97,000 are victims of alcohol-related sexual assault or date rape. A striking number of college students also report having experienced alcohol-induced memory blackouts. One recent study indicated that among nonabstaining college students, 40 percent reported experiencing a blackout within the past year, and

♣ **It's A Fact!!**
Epidemiology provides a profile of how specific populations of young people differ in their drinking patterns. Drinking, including heavy drinking, is common and accepted among college students, with consequences affecting both those who do the drinking and those who do not. Rates of heavy drinking among 18- to 25-year-olds in the military are much higher than among civilians. There is considerable variation between Whites and other ethnic/racial minority youth with respect to drinking, but also significant variation within these populations. Research is needed to determine how national origin, tribal affiliation, acculturation, immigration status, and language all influence drinking patterns among youth.

9.4 percent reported having a blackout within the past two weeks. This could relate to students' tendency to be unaware of standard drink volumes and to overpour drinks, thus underestimating their consumption. It is not known if younger drinkers are more susceptible to the memory-impairing effects of alcohol, but one study in humans showed that a dose of alcohol resulting in a BAC in the range of 80 mg/dl significantly disrupted learning in people in their early twenties but had little effect on people in their late twenties.

Drinking in college varies from campus to campus and from person to person. Levels and patterns of consumption are associated with individual, intracampus, and intercampus factors. For example, athletes and members of fraternities and sororities are among the heaviest drinkers on most campuses, and students in the northeast and on campuses where athletics and Greek organizations are prominent tend to drink more than their counterparts at other institutions.

Underage And Youthful Drinking Among Military Personnel

The Department of Defense (DOD) conducts periodic surveys to assess alcohol use and other health-related behaviors among military personnel. Approximately 193,000 of 1.4 million active duty military personnel are between the ages of 17 and 20. These surveys, therefore, provide important information about underage drinking in an important subset of young people.

- 33.3 percent of military personnel age 20 and younger are "abstainers" (drink once-a-year or less).

- 15.7 percent are "infrequent/light" drinkers (one to four drinks per typical occasion, one to three times per month).

- 10.4 percent are "moderate" drinkers (one drink per typical drinking occasion at least once a week, or two to four drinks per typical drinking occasion two to three times per month, or five or more drinks per typical drinking occasion once a month or less).

- 14.4 percent are "moderate/heavy" drinkers (two to four drinks per typical drinking occasion at least once a week or five or more drinks per typical drinking occasion two to three times per month).

- 26.1 percent are "heavy" drinkers (five or more drinks per typical drinking occasion at least once a week).

A comparison of data from the 2002 DOD survey with data from the 2001 National Household Survey on Drug Abuse (NHSDA)—in which heavy alcohol use is defined as five or more drinks on one occasion on five or more days in the past 30 days—indicates that rates of heavy drinking among 18- to 25-year-olds in the military are higher than for civilians of the same age (32.2 percent versus 17.8 percent for men, and 8.1 percent versus 5.5 percent for women).

The surveys conducted by the DOD also indicate that substantial numbers of youth in the military experience negative consequences from drinking. The 2002 data show that, during the 12 months prior to the survey, more than one-fifth of the most junior enlisted personnel (who typically are between the ages of 17 and 20) experienced serious consequences as a result of drinking or a drinking-related illness, including military punishment, alcohol-related arrest, and the need for detoxification, and that more than one-fourth experienced a productivity loss because of alcohol use. DOD investigators classified more than one-fifth of survey participants as alcohol "dependent" based on the number of days during the previous 12 months that they reported (1) withdrawal symptoms, (2) inability to recall things that happened while drinking, (3) inability to stop drinking before becoming drunk, or (4) morning drinking.

Minority Youth

According to national surveys, there is considerable variation between Whites and ethnic/racial minorities with respect to alcohol consumption. Minority youth generally start drinking at older ages than their White non-Hispanic counterparts. A greater difference also exists in levels of drinking between male and female minority youth and a greater percentage of minority youth abstain or drink very little. Although a "typical" pattern of underage drinking could never be attributed to any specific minority group, it is useful to compare minority groups to identify potential risk and protective factors that may be operating to produce some of the observed differences in drinking practices. With a burgeoning minority population, it is also essential to better understand these factors to help design and implement the most effective prevention and intervention programs.

Data from a recent nationwide survey reveal that about three-fourths of White, American Indian, and Hispanic high school seniors used alcohol in the past year. More than six percent of American Indian and five percent of Mexican and Cuban American seniors report daily drinking, compared with one percent to 3.8 percent for all other groups. The limited data on Hispanic and American Indian adults suggest that, among those who drink, there is a tendency toward high average intake per drinking day. Youth survey data suggest that some students establish a pattern of heavy drinking by their senior year of high school. About 60 percent of African American and about 57 percent of Asian American high school seniors report having used alcohol in the past 12 months, and about 32.5 percent in both groups report having used it in the past 30 days. However, there appears to be a "crossover" effect for African Americans. That is, even though they use less alcohol as youths than their non-Hispanic White counterparts, rates of heavy and problem drinking among African American adults, especially males, are higher than for non-Hispanic Whites.

Studies of race and ethnicity should be conducted with sufficiently large and diverse samples to allow investigators to assess variations in drinking by national origin or tribal affiliation, acculturation, immigration status, and language. Significant variation exists among Hispanics and among American Indians. Recent evidence indicates that members of some American Indian groups are more likely to abstain than are people in the general U.S. population. Like their Mexican American counterparts, American Indian drinkers, however, consume more alcohol per drinking occasion. In addition, although Asian Americans often are considered the "model minority," with low rates of alcohol use, most current literature does not include data from rapidly growing at-risk Asian groups such as Southeast Asians, Koreans, and Filipinos, or groups believed to have higher rates of alcohol use, such as Native Hawaiians and other Pacific Islanders.

Although there is clear evidence of genetic variability in alcohol metabolism, we have yet to fully understand the interplay of genetic and environmental variables. For example, the inability to metabolize alcohol efficiently, deemed a protective factor in a subset of the Asian population because of the unpleasant effects of drinking, often results in facial flushing. Highlighting the complexity of the interplay between genetic and environmental variables is the observation that Asian American drinking often increases with level of acculturation in spite of the flushing response.

Chapter 6

Underage Drinking: Adverse Consequences

What Is Underage Drinking?

When anyone under age 21 drinks alcohol, it is called underage drinking. And underage drinking is against the law, except in special cases, such as when it is part of a religious ceremony. Underage drinking is also dangerous. It can harm the mind and body of a growing teen in ways many people don't realize.

Yet, children and teens still drink, even though it can harm them. Underage drinking is a serious problem with roots deep in our culture. It is time to change that picture. It's time to take action. It's time to stop looking the other way.

Why Is Underage Drinking A Problem?

There are many reasons that underage drinking is a problem. Some of the reasons are listed below:

- So many young people drink. Many more young people use alcohol than tobacco or illegal drugs. By age 18, more than 70% of teens have had at least one drink.

About This Chapter: This chapter includes excerpts from "The Surgeon General's Call To Action To Prevent And Reduce Underage Drinking: What It Means to You," Office of the Surgeon General, U.S. Department of Health and Human Services, 2007.

- When young people drink, they drink a lot at one time. Teens drink less often than adults, but when teens do drink, they drink more than adults. On average, young people have about five drinks on a single occasion. This is called binge drinking—a very dangerous way of drinking that can lead to serious problems and even death.

> **♣ It's A Fact!!**
> Drinking alcohol can harm the growing body and brain. That's why it's important for young people to grow up alcohol-free.
>
> Source: Office of the Surgeon General, 2007.

- Early drinking can cause later alcohol problems. Of adults who started drinking before age 15, around 40% say they have the signs of alcohol dependence. That rate is four times higher than for adults who didn't drink until they were 21 years old.

- Alcohol may have a special appeal for young people. The teen years are a time of adventure, challenges, and taking risks. Alcohol is often one of the risks young people take. But most people don't know how alcohol affects a teen's body and behavior. They don't realize that alcohol can affect young people in different ways from adults. And they don't realize that underage drinkers can also harm people other than themselves.

The Results Of Underage Drinking Can Be Grave

Many people don't know that underage alcohol use can have dire consequences.

- It is a major cause of death from injuries among young people. Each year, approximately 5,000 people under the age of 21 die as a result of underage drinking; this includes about 1,900 deaths from motor vehicle crashes, 1,600 as a result of homicides, 300 from suicide, as well as hundreds from other injuries such as falls, burns, and drownings.

- It increases the risk of carrying out, or being a victim of, a physical or sexual assault and can affect the body in many ways. The effects of alcohol range from hangovers to death from alcohol poisoning.

- It can lead to other problems. These may include bad grades in school, run-ins with the law, and drug use.

- It affects how well a young person judges risk and makes sound decisions. For example, after drinking, a teen may see nothing wrong with driving a car or riding with a driver who has been drinking.

♣ It's A Fact!!

- In any month, more youth are drinking than are smoking cigarettes or using marijuana.

- As they grow older, the chance that young people will use alcohol grows. Approximately 10% of 12-year-olds say they have used alcohol at least once; by age 13, that number doubles; and by age 15, approximately 50% have had at least one drink.

- Alcohol dependence is a term doctors use when people have trouble controlling their drinking, and when their consumption of, or preoccupation with, alcohol occurs to the extent that it interferes with normal personal, family, social, or work life. Alcohol dependence rates are highest among young people between ages 18 and 20, when they're not even old enough to drink legally.

- The greatest influence on young people's decisions to begin drinking is the world they live in. This "world" includes their families, friends, schools, the larger community, and society as a whole.

- Alcohol use by young people often is made possible by adults. After all, teens can't legally get alcohol on their own.

- Most young people who start drinking before age 21 do so when they are about 13–14 years old. That's why it's important to start talking early and keep talking about underage drinking.

Source: Office of the Surgeon General, 2007.

- It plays a role in risky sexual activity. This can increase the chance of teen pregnancy and sexually transmitted diseases (STDs), including human immunodeficiency virus (HIV), the virus that causes acquired immune deficiency syndrome (AIDS).

- It can harm the growing brain, especially when teens drink a lot. Today we know that the brain continues to develop from birth, through the teen years, and into the mid-twenties.

The Teen Years Are A Time Of Many Changes

The teen years are a time of accelerated change—both physical and emotional change.

- Boys physically become young men and girls become young women.

- Young people move from elementary to middle to high school. Responsibilities increase. For example, teens learn to drive, may get a job, have more chores, and more homework.

- Teens spend less time with their parents. They spend more time alone or with friends. They also like to stay up later and sleep in.

- Teens search for who they really are and who they want to be. They worry about friendships, social groups, and they have growing romantic and sexual interests.

- The desire for adventure, excitement, and action increases. That's why many young people want to take more chances, try new things, and be more independent.

> ✤ **It's A Fact!!**
> Rates of death and injury nearly triple between the early teen years and early adult life. Dangerous activities like underage drinking play a large role. That's why ending teen alcohol use can help save lives.
>
> Source: Office of the Surgeon General, 2007.

These changes are important steps on the road to adult life. However, these changes also increase the chance that some young people may turn to alcohol.

♣ **It's A Fact!!**

Most middle school students don't drink. But some do, and this can lead to serious troubles. By drinking too much at any age, people can dig themselves into holes of trouble. Some dig faster than others and have problems more quickly. They can lose friends, fall behind at school or work, cause family tension, harm their health, and bring on money problems, as you can see below.

- **Losing Friends:** Friends start pulling back or drifting away. Only friends who are heavy drinkers will remain.

- **Problems At Work Or At School:** Being late, missing days, not working up to abilities, and putting off responsibilities are just a few of the problems. Falling behind comes first, which can lead to losing a job or failing school.

- **Tension Builds Up In The Family:** Homes with heavy drinkers have less fun and closeness, more arguments, and higher rates of divorce and child abuse.

- **Fitness And Health:** Heavy drinking can weaken the heart muscle and contribute to weight gain. It can also cause many other serious, life-threatening health problems, including addiction.

- **Money Problems:** Troubles with money grow when too much is spent on alcohol and on paying for problems or poor decisions caused by drinking.

Since alcohol can cloud a person's judgment, heavy drinkers often feel misunderstood, unfairly treated, harassed, or just plain unlucky. As things get worse they may be more likely to drink, and dig their holes even deeper.

It's easy to see why using alcohol as a solution to problems, or a way of trying to cope, is trouble. Drinking should never take the place of talking things through and working out difficulties in other ways.

Source: "Too Much, Too Soon, Too Risky," National Institute on Alcohol Abuse and Alcoholism (http://www.thecoolspot.gov), 2004.

The different "worlds" teens live in can have a big effect on their drinking. Some young people are more involved with family than others. Others turn to their friends first. Still others turn to social groups like sports teams and clubs, faith-based groups, or groups of like-minded youth. The internet, media, music, and videos are also an important part of the world of most teens. All of these influences affect a young person's choices about using alcohol.

Why Some Teens Choose To Drink

Many things affect a young person's decisions about drinking.

- The different "worlds" in which teens live, including family, friends, school, and community

- A greater desire to take risks

- Less connection to parents and more independence

- More time spent with friends and by themselves

- Increased stress

- Greater attention to what they see and hear about alcohol

Teens With Behavior Or Family Problems Are At Higher Risk For Alcohol Use

If anyone in the family has a drinking problem, it can affect the entire family. It also may affect a teen's choices about drinking.

Also, youth with histories of behavior problems (for example, delinquent activity, impulsive actions, and difficulty controlling responses) are more likely to use alcohol than are other young people. The same is true for youth that have an unusually strong desire for new experiences and sensations and for those with histories of family conflict, stress, and/or alcohol problems.

Underage Drinking Is Everyone's Problem

Underage drinking can affect anyone, including people who don't drink.

- Underage alcohol use can lead to dangerous behavior, property damage, and violence.

- The results can be injury and even death for the drinker and for other people nearby.

- About 45% of people who die in car crashes involving a drinking driver under age 21 are people other than the driver.

The effects of underage drinking can be felt by everyone. That makes underage alcohol use everyone's problem.

Changing Attitudes About Underage Drinking

It's time to change how we all think, talk, and act when it comes to underage drinking. We need to stop accepting it and to start discouraging it. It's time for young people to understand that it is not okay for them to drink alcohol. Ending underage drinking is everyone's job.

- Everyone can work together to create a community where young people can grow up and feel good about themselves without drinking.

- Everyone in the community should deliver the message that underage drinking is not okay. The message should be the same whether youth hear it in school, at home, in places of worship, on the sports field, in youth programs, or in other places where young people gather.

- Families can help prevent underage drinking by staying involved in their children's lives. It is important for families to pay attention to what's happening with their teens.

- Young people can learn about the dangers of alcohol use. They can change how they and others think about drinking.

What Communities Can Do About Underage Drinking

Underage alcohol use is not inevitable. It will take everyone in the community to make change happen. All of us can help change attitudes about teen drinking and help replace environments that enable underage alcohol use with environments that discourage it.

After all, changing how people think isn't easy. Drinking is legal for adults. That's why some people think drinking is a rite of passage for youth. Many young people think drinking is a way for them to feel more grown up. People of all ages forget that underage drinking is illegal and dangerous.

Communities can come together to encourage a new attitude about underage drinking. A community that opposes underage drinking can help change how people think and act. But it takes time. So it's important to keep sending the message that the community does not approve of underage drinking. Together, communities can support teen decisions not to drink.

Get Organized

- Work on underage drinking as a community health and safety problem that everyone can solve together.

- Organize groups to change community thinking about underage alcohol use. Support the message that underage drinking is not okay.

- Work with sponsors of community events to help them send the message that underage drinking is not allowed.

Share Knowledge

- Get the word out about policies to prevent underage drinking. This includes age checks for people buying alcohol, including on the internet.

- Help people learn about the latest research on underage alcohol use. Include information about the dangers of youth alcohol use for teens and others. An informed public is key to ending underage drinking.

- Teach young people about the dangers of underage alcohol use. Support programs that help teens already involved with drinking.

Change The Teen Scene

- Create friendly, alcohol-free places where teens can gather.

- Create programs, including volunteer work, where young people can grow, explore their options, succeed, and feel good about themselves without alcohol.

- Help teens realize that underage drinking is unhealthy and can drastically impact their lives like "doing drugs" or smoking.

- Let teens involved with underage drinking know that it's okay to ask for and get help.

Take Action

- Work to change community attitudes about underage drinking.

- Focus as much community attention on underage drinking as on tobacco and drug use.

- Work with state, tribal, and local groups to reduce underage drinking.

- Make it easier for young people who are involved with—or at risk for—underage drinking to get help.

- Get the word out about underage drinking laws. The law that makes drinking under age 21 illegal is only one of them. Other laws forbid selling or giving alcohol to youth. Others make it against the law to drink and drive. Work to help ensure these laws are always enforced.

☞ Remember!!

The legal drinking age is 21, and underage drinking can be a threat to health and development.

Source: Office of the Surgeon General, 2007.

Part Two

Alcohol's Effect On The Body

Chapter 7

The Physical Effects Of Alcohol On Your Body

Alcohol is a drug. It can cause short-term and long-term damage to your body.

How can alcohol hurt your body?

- **Brain:** Drinking alcohol leads to a loss of coordination, poor judgment, slowed reflexes, distorted vision, loss of memory, and even blackouts.

- **Heart:** Drinking alcohol could cause your blood pressure to rise, increase your heart rate, cause your heart to beat abnormally, and can increase the size of your heart.

- **Stomach:** You're putting empty calories into your body, which could cause weight gain. If you drink too much, you may vomit because alcohol is toxic. Drinking alcohol can also cause stomach ulcers and cancer.

- **Liver:** Drinking alcohol could cause diseases such as cirrhosis (pronounced: sir-o-sis). It can also cause hepatitis (inflamed liver) or even liver cancer, which weakens the liver's ability to clot and keep our blood free from poisons and bacteria.

About This Chapter: Excerpted from "Straight Talk about Alcohol," National Women's Health Information Center (www.4girls.gov), March 2008.

- **Reproductive System:** Heavy drinking can cause painful periods, heavy flow, discomfort before your period (PMS), and irregular periods (not getting your period when you're supposed to). Drinking also raises the risk of getting sexually assaulted and having unsafe sex.

How much alcohol would it take to affect a person?

Every person is affected differently by alcohol. Females have less body water than males. With less water, alcohol reaches a girl's organs faster than a guy's. Other factors that affect how fast you process alcohol are your weight, how much you've eaten, and how fast you drink. Your hormones also affect alcohol absorption. During the month, your hormones go up and down, which changes how much alcohol stays in your blood.

Remember that you don't have to slur words or stumble around to be impaired or intoxicated (drunk). Once you have been impaired or intoxicated, the only thing that will sober you up is time. Coffee, cold showers, exercise, or other things you've heard about will not speed up your body's rate of getting rid of alcohol from your system.

♣ **It's A Fact!!**
The Effects Of Hangover

Although not traditionally thought of as a medical problem, a review of studies found that hangovers have significant consequences that include changes in liver function, hormonal balance, and mental functioning and an increased risk for depression and cardiac events. Hangovers can impair job performance, increasing the risk for mistakes and accidents. Interestingly, hangovers are generally more common in light-to-moderate drinkers than heavy and chronic drinkers, suggesting that binge drinking can be as threatening as chronic drinking. Any man who drinks more than five drinks or any woman who has more than three drinks is at risk for a hangover.

Source: Excerpted from "Alcoholism," © 2007 A.D.A.M., Inc. Reprinted with permission.

♣ It's A Fact!!

Sensitivity To The Effects Of Alcohol Use

Animal research indicates that adolescents in general are more sensitive than adults to the stimulating effects of alcohol and less sensitive to some of the aversive effects of acute alcohol intoxication, such as sedation, hangover, and ataxia (loss of muscular coordination). This difference in sensitivity between adolescents and adults may make adolescents more vulnerable to certain harmful effects of alcohol use. For example, adolescents are able to drink more than adults—who might pass out or be inclined to go to sleep. Adolescents are also more likely than adults to initiate activities when they are too impaired to perform them competently, such as driving, and also are more likely to drink to the point of coma. Furthermore, in the case of driving, each drink increases impairment more for adolescents than adult, and children with alcoholic parents may be at even greater risk for excessive drinking resulting from a combination of genetic and developmental factors that lower sensitivity to alcohol.

Source: From *The Surgeon General's Call To Action To Prevent And Reduce Underage Drinking*, Office of the Surgeon General, U.S. Department of Health and Human Services, 2007.

What exactly do "impaired" and "intoxicated" mean?

Whether you are impaired or intoxicated depends on how much alcohol is in your body. The amount of alcohol in your body is measured in terms of blood alcohol content (BAC), or the number of grams of alcohol in 100 millimeters of blood. BAC can be measured in blood, urine, or breath. Impairment and intoxication are defined as follows:

- Impairment starts with your first drink. It's when the amount of alcohol you have had affects your judgment, coordination, and reaction time. With low BAC levels, some people may not appear to be impaired, but they have been affected. Since it takes time for alcohol to leave the stomach and enter the blood stream, a person may continue to become more impaired for a period of time following their last drink.

♣ It's A Fact!!

There's no question that years of heavy drinking can seriously damage health and even kill. But some of the dangers won't wait. They are right in the here and now.

That's because alcohol can harm judgment, coordination, and reflexes. It can cause people to lose control, take chances, and do things they never would do otherwise.

As a result, teens who drink can be injured or killed, even the first time they try alcohol. In fact, alcohol is linked with an estimated 5,000 deaths in people under age 21 each year—more than all illegal drugs combined.

- **Deadly Car Crashes:** Motor vehicle crashes are the leading cause of death in people aged 15 to 20. Deadly crashes involving alcohol are twice as common in teens compared with people 21 and older. That's because teens are not as experienced with driving, and their judgment skills are harmed more by alcohol, even if they drink less than adults.

- **Drowning And Other Deaths:** Mixing drinking with swimming or boating can be fatal. Four out of 10 teens who drown have been drinking alcohol. Underage drinking has also been linked with deaths and injuries from burns, falls, alcohol poisoning, and suicide.

Will others survive?

Drinking teens not only risk hurting themselves. They risk hurting their friends, family, and people they have never even met. Drinking teens, who drive, are more likely than adults to kill someone else, whether it's passengers in their cars, people in other cars, or pedestrians.

Source: "Too Much, Too Soon, Too Risky," an undated document produced by the National Institute on Alcohol Abuse and Alcoholism, http://www.thecoolspot.gov; accessed November 2008.

• Intoxication is a legal term. Anyone who is found with a BAC level at or above the intoxication limit is breaking the law and can be punished. It normally doesn't take many drinks to reach that level!

What about my parents? They drink and it doesn't seem to hurt them.

Adults process alcohol differently than teens. Because their bodies are mature, adults can handle alcohol as long as they drink a reasonable amount. Teens, however, are still growing in many ways, so even a small amount of alcohol can affect their physical and mental development. Besides, your parents are allowed by law to drink. When they drink, they should be doing it responsibly and in moderation—which means they never drive after drinking, and they have one to two drinks a day or less. So it's okay if they have a glass of wine at dinner or a beer during the football game. But if your parents misuse alcohol for any period of time, they will also cause serious damage to their health.

Chapter 8

Understanding Blood Alcohol Concentration

What is blood alcohol concentration (BAC)?

The amount of alcohol in a person's body is measured by the weight of the alcohol in a certain volume of blood. This is called the blood alcohol concentration, or BAC.

Alcohol is absorbed directly through the walls of the stomach and the small intestine, goes into the bloodstream, and travels throughout the body and to the brain.

Alcohol is quickly absorbed and can be measured within 30 to 70 minutes after a person has had a drink.

Does the type of alcohol I drink affect my BAC?

No. A drink is a drink, is a drink.

A typical drink equals about half an ounce of alcohol (.54 ounces, to be exact). This is the approximate amount of alcohol found in one shot of distilled spirits, or one 5-ounce glass of wine, or one 12-ounce beer.

About This Chapter: From "The ABCs of BAC," National Highway Traffic Safety Administration (NHTSA), February 2005.

What about other medications or drugs?

Medications or drugs will not change your BAC. However, if you drink alcohol while taking certain medications, you may feel—and be—more impaired, which can affect your ability to perform driving-related tasks.

When am I impaired?

Because of the multitude of factors that affect BAC, it is very difficult to assess your own BAC or impairment. Though small amounts of alcohol affect one's brain and the ability to drive, people often swear they are "fine" after several drinks—but in fact, the failure to recognize alcohol impairment is often a symptom of impairment.

Table 8.1. Common Symptoms People Exhibit At Various BAC Levels

The following chart contains some of the more common symptoms people exhibit at various BAC levels and the probable effects on driving ability.

Blood Alcohol Concentration (BAC)	Typical Effects	Predictable Effects on Driving
.02%	Some loss of judgment; Relaxation; Slight body warmth; Altered mood	Decline in visual functions (rapid tracking of a moving target); Decline in ability to perform two tasks at the same time (divided attention)
.05%	Exaggerated behavior; May have loss of small-muscle control (for example, focusing your eyes); Impaired judgment; Usually good feeling; Lowered alertness; Release of inhibition	Reduced coordination; Reduced ability to track moving objects; Difficulty steering; Reduced response to emergency driving situations

While the lower stages of alcohol impairment are undetectable to others, the drinker knows vaguely when the "buzz" begins. A person will likely be too impaired to drive before looking—or maybe even feeling—"drunk."

How will I know I'm impaired, and why should I care?

Alcohol steadily decreases a person's ability to drive a motor vehicle safely. The more you drink, the greater the effect. As with BAC, the signs of impairment differ with the individual.

In single-vehicle crashes, the relative risk of a driver with BAC between .08 and .10 is at least 11 times greater than for drivers with a BAC of zero, and 52 times greater for young males. Further, many studies have

Table 8.1. Continued

BAC	Typical Effects	Predictable Effects on Driving
.08%	Muscle coordination becomes poor (for example, balance, speech, vision, reaction time, and hearing); Harder to detect danger; Judgment, self-control, reasoning, and memory are impaired	Concentration; Short-term memory loss; Speed control; Reduced information processing capability (for example, signal detection, visual search); Impaired perception
.10%	Clear deterioration of reaction time and control; Slurred speech, poor coordination, and slowed thinking	Reduced ability to maintain lane position and brake appropriately
.15%	Far less muscle control than normal; Vomiting may occur (unless this level is reached slowly or a person has developed a tolerance for alcohol; Major loss of balance	Substantial impairment in vehicle control, attention to driving task, and in necessary visual and auditory information processing

Source: National Highway Traffic Safety Administration, February 2005.

shown that even small amounts of alcohol can impair a person's ability to drive.

Every state has passed a law making it illegal to drive with a BAC of .08 or higher. A driver can also be arrested with a BAC below .08 when a law enforcement officer has probable cause, based on the driver's behavior.

♣ It's A Fact!!
What affects my blood alcohol concentration (BAC)?

How fast a person's BAC rises varies with a number of factors.

- **The Number Of Drinks:** The more you drink, the higher the BAC.

- **How Fast You Drink:** When alcohol is consumed quickly, you will reach a higher BAC than when it is consumed over a longer period of time.

- **Your Gender:** Women generally have less water and more body fat per pound of body weight than men. Alcohol does not go into fat cells as easily as other cells, so more alcohol remains in the blood of women.

- **Your Weight:** The more you weigh, the more water is present in your body. This water dilutes the alcohol and lowers the BAC.

- **Food In Your Stomach:** Absorption will be slowed if you've had something to eat.

Source: National Highway Traffic Safety Administration, February 2005.

What can I do to stay safe when I plan on drinking?

Teens should not drink alcohol, but if you plan on drinking, plan not to drive.

- Choose a non-drinking friend as a designated driver.

- Ask ahead of time if you can stay over at your host's house.

- Take a taxi (your community may have a Safe Rides program for a free ride home).

- Always wear your safety belt—it's your best defense against impaired drivers.

Chapter 9

Alcohol Intoxication And Alcohol Poisoning

What Is Intoxication?

Intoxication Occurs Long Before Someone Passes Out

Intoxication is the point at which alcohol depresses the central nervous system so that mood and physical and mental abilities are noticeably changed. Each person responds somewhat differently to the effects of alcohol based on mood, the drinking setting, physical health, and tolerance for the chemical. Tolerance, however, is completely unrelated to a person's blood alcohol content (BAC). BAC is the amount of alcohol in one's system based on weight, number of drinks, and the period of time during which alcohol is consumed. The legal definition of intoxication is a BAC of .08. It is suggested that a person not exceed a BAC of .056, as this is the point where the positive, relaxed, euphoric effects of the alcohol are experienced. When a BAC of .056 is exceeded, the negative, depressant effects of alcohol take place.

A BAC of .06 to .10 is considered the point of diminishing returns. Typically a person at this BAC will experience the following:

About This Chapter: This chapter includes information from "What is Intoxication?" © 2008 University of Notre Dame Office of Alcohol and Drug Education (www.oade.nd.edu). Reprinted with permission. Additional information is from "Facts About Alcohol Poisoning," National Institute on Alcohol Abuse and Alcoholism (NIAAA), July 2007.

Table 9.1. Blood Alcohol Content (BAC) Level Generalized Dose Specific Effects

BAC Level	Effect Of Alcohol
BAC = 0.02 to 0.03%	No loss of coordination, slight euphoria, and loss of shyness. Depressant effects are not apparent.
BAC = 0.04 to 0.06%	Feeling of well-being, relaxation, lower inhibitions, and sensation of warmth. Euphoria. Some minor impairment of reasoning and memory, lowering of caution.
BAC = 0.07 to 0.09%	Slight impairment of balance, speech, vision, reaction time, and hearing. Euphoria. Reduced judgment and self-control. Impaired reasoning, memory, and sense of cautiousness.
BAC = 0.10-0.125%	Significant impairment of motor coordination and loss of good judgment. Speech may be slurred; balance, vision, reaction time, and hearing will be impaired.
BAC = 0.13-0.15%	Gross motor impairment and lack of physical control. Blurred vision and major loss of balance. Euphoria is reducing and dysphoria is beginning to appear.
BAC = 0.16-0.20%	Dysphoria predominates, nausea may appear. The drinker has the appearance of a "sloppy drunk." May vomit.
BAC = 0.25%	Needs assistance in walking; total mental confusion. Dysphoria with nausea and some vomiting. Death has occurred at this level, and it is considered a medical emergency.
BAC = 0.30%	Loss of consciousness.
BAC = 0.40% +	Onset of coma, possible death due to respiratory arrest.

Source: © 2008 University of Notre Dame Office of Alcohol and Drug Education (OADE).

- Impaired judgment, inappropriate behavior (such as drinking competitively or annoying others)

- Impaired coordination (stumbling, swaying, staggering, or loss of fine motor skills; distance acuity, glare recovery)

- Slurred speech, talkative

- Diminished of senses (speaks louder; cannot hear as well as normal; vision is not as clear; glassy, unfocused eyes)

- Slowed mental processing (can only do one task at a time, forgetting things, lighting more than one cigarette at a time, or losing their train of thought, cannot listen well, follow conversations well, or understand what others are saying)

- Intensified emotions (overly friendly, laughing intensely, displaying mood swings)

- Lowered Inhibitions

Some people may become significantly more affected at lower blood alcohol levels, whereas others at similar BACs may not appear to show symptoms due to developed tolerance. Table 9.1 indicates the typical effects experienced at varying blood alcohol levels.

Remember, there are no absolutes.

Facts About Alcohol Poisoning

Excessive drinking can be hazardous to everyone's health. It can be particularly stressful if you are the sober one taking care of your friend who is vomiting while you are trying to study for an exam.

Some people laugh at the behavior of others who are drunk. Some think it's even funnier when they pass out. But there is nothing funny about the aspiration of vomit leading to asphyxiation or the poisoning of the respiratory center in the brain, both of which can result in death.

Do you know about the dangers of alcohol poisoning or when should you seek professional help for a friend? Sadly enough, too many students say

✤ It's A Fact!!

Factors That Affect Intoxication

- **Food:** Always eat before drinking, especially foods high in protein. Having food in your stomach will help slow down the processing of alcohol.

- **Strength Of Drink:** Stronger drinks will result in higher blood alcohol concentration. Understand drink equivalents.

- **Body Weight/Body Type:** The less you weigh, the more you will be affected by a given amount of alcohol. For people of the same weight, individuals with a lower percentage of body fat will have lower blood alcohol contents (BACs) than those with a higher percentage of body fat.

- **Gender:** Women have less of the enzyme dehydrogenase that breaks down alcohol in the stomach. Hormone levels also affect the body's ability to process alcohol women will experience a higher BAC before menstruation on the same amount of alcohol they usually drink. Women tend to have a higher percentage of body fat and a lower percentage of water.

- **Rate Of Consumption:** The faster a person consumes drinks, the quicker the blood alcohol concentration will rise.

- **Functional Tolerance:** Functional tolerance is a decrease in the body's sensitivity to alcohol's effects. In other words, a person exhibiting functional tolerance will not seem to be as intoxicated as a person with little or no functional tolerance. This is a behavioral adaptation to the effects of alcohol, and as long as the liver continues to eliminate alcohol at the rate of one drink per hour, it will have no effect on blood alcohol concentration.

- **Medications:** Most medications do have some type of reaction when mixed with alcohol, always consult with your physician before mixing any medication with alcohol.

- **Illness:** If you are sick there is a good chance you are dehydrated. This will result in a higher blood alcohol concentration. Dehydration can also make your liver less efficient at eliminating alcohol.

- **Fatigue:** Fatigue causes many of the same symptoms as intoxication. If you are fatigued before drinking, intoxication will intensify the symptoms.

Source: © 2008 University of Notre Dame Office of Alcohol and Drug Education (OADE).

they wish they had sought medical treatment for a friend. Many end up feeling responsible for alcohol-related tragedies that could have easily been prevented.

Common myths about sobering up include drinking black coffee, taking a cold bath or shower, sleeping it off, or walking it off. But these are just myths, and they don't work. The only thing that reverses the effects of alcohol is time—something you may not have if you are suffering from alcohol poisoning. And many different factors affect the level of intoxication of an individual, so it's difficult to gauge exactly how much is too much.

♣ It's A Fact!!
Critical Signs for Alcohol Poisoning

- Mental confusion, stupor, coma, or person cannot be roused

- Vomiting

- Seizures

- Slow breathing (fewer than eight breaths per minute)

- Irregular breathing (10 seconds or more between breaths)

- Hypothermia (low body temperature), bluish skin color, paleness

Source: National Institute on Alcohol Abuse and Alcoholism (NIAAA), July 2007.

What Happens To Your Body When You Get Alcohol Poisoning?

Alcohol depresses nerves that control involuntary actions such as breathing and the gag reflex (which prevents choking). A fatal dose of alcohol will eventually stop these functions.

It is common for someone who drinks excessive alcohol to vomit since alcohol is an irritant to the stomach. There is then the danger of choking on vomit, which could cause death by asphyxiation in a person who is not conscious because of intoxication.

You should also know that a person's blood alcohol concentration (BAC) can continue to rise even while he or she is passed out. Even after a person stops drinking, alcohol in the stomach and intestine continues to enter the bloodstream and circulate throughout the body. It is dangerous to assume the person will be fine by sleeping it off.

What Should I Do If I Suspect Someone Has Alcohol Poisoning?

- Know the danger signals.

- Do not wait for all symptoms to be present.

- Be aware that a person who has passed out may die.

- If there is any suspicion of an alcohol overdose, call 911 for help. Don't try to guess the level of drunkenness.

What Can Happen To Someone With Alcohol Poisoning That Goes Untreated?

- Victim chokes on his or her own vomit.

- Breathing slows, becomes irregular, or stops.

- Heart beats irregularly or stops.

- Hypothermia (low body temperature).

- Hypoglycemia (too little blood sugar) leads to seizures.

- Untreated severe dehydration from vomiting can cause seizures, permanent brain damage, or death.

> ### ✎ What's It Mean?
>
> Intoxication: A synonym for poisoning.
>
> Poison: Any substance, either taken internally or applied externally, that is injurious to health or dangerous to life.
>
> Poisoning: The administering of poison (a synonym for intoxication); the state of being poisoned.
>
> Source: From *Stedman's Medical Dictionary, 27th Edition*, copyright © 2000 Lippincott Williams & Wilkins. All rights reserved.

Even if the victim lives, an alcohol overdose can lead to irreversible brain damage. Rapid binge drinking (which often happens on a bet or a dare) is especially dangerous because the victim can ingest a fatal dose before becoming unconscious.

Don't be afraid to seek medical help for a friend who has had too much to drink. Don't worry that your friend may become angry or embarrassed—remember, you cared enough to help. Always be safe, not sorry.

Chapter 10

Alcohol And The Brain

Alcohol's Damaging Effects On The Brain

Difficulty walking, blurred vision, slurred speech, slowed reaction times, impaired memory—clearly, alcohol affects the brain. Some of these impairments are detectable after only one or two drinks and quickly resolve when drinking stops. On the other hand, a person who drinks heavily over a long period of time may have brain deficits that persist well after he or she achieves sobriety. Exactly how alcohol affects the brain and the likelihood of reversing the impact of heavy drinking on the brain remain hot topics in alcohol research today.

We do know that heavy drinking may have extensive and far-reaching effects on the brain, ranging from simple "slips" in memory to permanent and debilitating conditions that require lifetime custodial care. And even moderate drinking leads to short-term impairment, as shown by extensive research on the impact of drinking on driving.

A number of factors influence how and to what extent alcohol affects the brain.

• How much and how often a person drinks

About This Chapter: This chapter includes excerpts from "Alcohol Alert: Alcohol's Damaging Effects On The Brain," National Institute on Alcohol Abuse and Alcoholism (NIAAA), October 2004.

- The age at which he or she first began drinking, and how long he or she has been drinking

- The person's age, level of education, gender, genetic background, and family history of alcoholism

- Whether he or she is at risk as a result of prenatal alcohol exposure

- His or her general health status

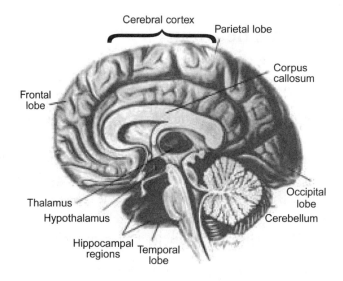

Figure 10.1. Schematic drawing of the human brain, showing regions vulnerable to alcoholism-related abnormalities.

Brain Damage From Other Causes

People who have been drinking large amounts of alcohol for long periods of time run the risk of developing serious and persistent changes in the brain. Damage may be a result of the direct effects of alcohol on the brain or may result indirectly, from a poor general health status or from severe liver disease.

For example, thiamine deficiency is a common occurrence in people with alcoholism and results from poor overall nutrition. Thiamine, also known as vitamin B1, is an essential nutrient required by all tissues, including the brain.

Thiamine is found in foods such as meat and poultry; whole grain cereals; nuts; and dried beans, peas, and soybeans. Many foods in the United States commonly are fortified with thiamine, including breads and cereals. As a result, most people consume sufficient amounts of thiamine in their diets. The typical intake for most Americans is two milligrams per day, and the recommended daily allowance (RDA) is 1.2 milligrams per day for men and 1.1 milligrams per day for women.

Wernicke–Korsakoff Syndrome

Up to 80 percent of alcoholics, however, have a deficiency in thiamine, and some of these people will go on to develop serious brain disorders such as Wernicke–Korsakoff syndrome (WKS). WKS is a disease that consists of two separate syndromes; a short-lived and severe condition called Wernicke's encephalopathy and a long-lasting and debilitating condition known as Korsakoff's psychosis.

The symptoms of Wernicke's encephalopathy include mental confusion, paralysis of the nerves that move the eyes, and difficulty with muscle coordination. For example, patients with Wernicke's encephalopathy may be too confused to find their way out of a room or may not even be able to walk. Many Wernicke's encephalopathy patients, however, do not exhibit all three of these signs and symptoms, and clinicians working with alcoholics must be aware that this disorder may be present even if the patient shows only one or two of them. In fact, studies performed after death indicate that many cases of thiamine deficiency-related encephalopathy may not be diagnosed in life because not all the "classic" signs and symptoms were present or recognized.

Approximately 80 to 90 percent of alcoholics with Wernicke's encephalopathy also develop Korsakoff's psychosis, a chronic and debilitating syndrome characterized by persistent learning and memory problems. Patients with Korsakoff's psychosis are forgetful and quickly frustrated and have difficulty with walking and coordination. Although these patients have problems remembering old information, it is their difficulty in "laying down" new information that is the most striking. For example, these patients can discuss in detail an event in their lives, but an hour later might not remember ever having the conversation.

Liver Disease

Most people realize that heavy, long-term drinking can damage the liver—the organ chiefly responsible for breaking down alcohol into harmless byproducts and clearing it from the body. But people may not be aware that prolonged liver dysfunction, such as liver cirrhosis resulting from excessive alcohol consumption, can harm the brain, leading to a serious and potentially fatal brain disorder known as hepatic encephalopathy.

♣ It's A Fact!!

The human brain is like a command center for the body. It alerts body parts and organs when something should happen and how to react. It only takes about 30 seconds for the first amounts of alcohol to reach the brain after ingestion. Once there, alcohol acts primarily on nerve cells deep in the brain.

The most highly developed part of the brain is the cerebral cortex, which encompasses about two-thirds of the brain mass and lies over and around most of the remaining structures of the brain. It is responsible for thinking, reasoning, perceiving, and producing and understanding language. The cerebral cortex is divided into specific areas involved in vision, hearing, touch, movement, and smell. The nerves in these parts of the brain talk to each other by electrical impulses that are enabled by neurotransmitters.

Alcohol acts as a depressant to the central nervous system and causes some neurotransmitters to become inhibited. Judgement and coordination, two processes of the central nervous system, become impaired.

Heavy drinking can inhibit the firing of the nerve cells that control breathing, a condition known as respiratory depression. This condition can be fatal. Even if the inhibition of the respiratory nerve cells does not cause death, drinking excessive alcohol may cause vomiting. When drunk and unconscious, a person may inhale fluids that have been vomited, resulting in death by asphyxiation.

Research now shows that significant brain development continues through adolescence. Therefore, alcohol may have quite different toxic effects on adolescent brains than on those of adults. Heavy alcohol use can impair brain function in adolescents, and it is unclear at present whether the damage is reversible.

Source: Excerpted from "Interactive Body," National Institute on Alcohol Abuse and Alcoholism (www.collegedrinkingprevention.gov), July 11, 2007.

> ♣ It's
> A Fact!!
> **Alcohol And
> The Maturing Brain**
>
> Research shows that the brain continues to develop throughout adolescence and well into young adulthood. Many scientists are concerned that drinking during this critical developmental period may lead to lifelong impairments in brain function, particularly as it relates to memory, motor skills, and coordination. Young adults are particularly likely to binge drink and to suffer repeated bouts of withdrawal from alcohol. (NIAAA defines binge drinking as consuming about four drinks for men or three drinks for women in about two hours.) This repeated withdrawal may be a key reason for alcohol's harmful effects on the brain.
>
> Even though research shows that drinking early in life can lead to impairment of brain function in adulthood, findings also show that not all young people who drink heavily or become alcohol dependent will experience the same level of impairment, and some may not show any damage at all. This is because factors such as genetics, drinking patterns, and the use of other drugs also influence risk.
>
> Source: "Alcohol Alert: Young Adult Drinking," National Institute on Alcohol Abuse and Alcoholism (NIAAA), April 2006.

Hepatic encephalopathy can cause changes in sleep patterns, mood, and personality; psychiatric conditions such as anxiety and depression; severe cognitive effects such as shortened attention span; and problems with coordination such as a flapping or shaking of the hands (called asterixis). In the most serious cases, patients may slip into a coma, which can be fatal.

New imaging techniques have enabled researchers to study specific brain regions in patients with alcoholic liver disease, giving them a better understanding of how hepatic encephalopathy develops. These studies have confirmed that at least two toxic substances, ammonia and manganese, have a role in the development of hepatic encephalopathy. Alcohol-damaged liver cells allow excess amounts of these harmful byproducts to enter the brain, thus harming brain cells.

Alcohol And The Developing Brain

Drinking during pregnancy can lead to a range of physical, learning, and behavioral effects in the developing brain, the most serious of which is a collection of symptoms known as fetal alcohol syndrome

♣ It's A Fact!!
Using High-Tech Tools To Assess Alcoholic Brain Damage

Researchers studying the effects of alcohol use on the brain are aided by advanced technology such as magnetic resonance imaging (MRI), diffusion tensor imaging (DTI), positron emission tomography (PET), and electrophysiological brain mapping. These tools are providing valuable insight into how alcohol affects the brain's structure and function.

Long-term heavy drinking may lead to shrinking of the brain and deficiencies in the fibers (white matter) that carry information between brain cells (gray matter). MRI and DTI are being used together to assess the brains of patients when they first stop chronic heavy drinking and again after long periods of sobriety, to monitor for possible relapse to drinking.

Memory formation and retrieval are highly influenced by factors such as attention and motivation. Studies using MRI are helping scientists to determine how memory and attention improve with long-time abstinence from alcohol, as well as what changes take place when a patient begins drinking again. The goal of these studies is to determine which alcohol-induced effects on the brain are permanent and which ones can be reversed with abstinence.

PET imaging is allowing researchers to visualize, in the living brain, the damage that results from heavy alcohol consumption. This "snapshot" of the brain's function enables scientists to analyze alcohol's effects on various nerve cell communication systems as well as on brain cell metabolism and blood flow within the brain. These studies have detected deficits in alcoholics, particularly in the frontal lobes, which are responsible for numerous functions associated with learning and memory, as well as in the cerebellum, which controls movement and coordination. PET also is a promising tool for monitoring the effects of alcoholism treatment and abstinence on damaged portions of the brain and may help in developing new medications to correct the chemical deficits found in the brains of people with alcohol dependence.

Another high-tech tool, electroencephalography (EEG), records the brain's electrical signals. Small electrodes are placed on the scalp to detect this electrical activity, which then is magnified and graphed as brain waves. These brain waves show real-time activity as it happens in the brain.

Source: NIAAA, October 2004.

(FAS). Children with FAS may have distinct facial features including skin folds at the corner of the eye, a low nasal bridge, a short nose, indistinct philtrum (the groove between the nose and upper lip), small head circumference, small eye openings, small midface, and a thin upper lip. FAS infants also are markedly smaller than average. Their brains may have less volume (microencephaly). And, they may have fewer numbers of brain cells (neurons) or fewer neurons that are able to function correctly, leading to long-term problems in learning and behavior.

Growing New Brain Cells

For decades scientists believed that the number of nerve cells in the adult brain was fixed early in life. If brain damage occurred, then, the best way to treat it was by strengthening the existing neurons, as new ones could not be added. In the 1960s, however, researchers found that new neurons are indeed generated in adulthood—a process called neurogenesis. These new cells originate from stem cells, which are cells that can divide indefinitely, renew themselves, and give rise to a variety of cell types. The discovery of brain stem cells and adult neurogenesis provides a new way of approaching the problem of alcohol-related changes in the brain and may lead to a clearer understanding of how best to treat and cure alcoholism.

For example, studies with animals show that high doses of alcohol lead to a disruption in the growth of new brain cells, and scientists believe it may be this lack of new growth that results in the long-term deficits found in key areas of the brain. Understanding how alcohol interacts with brain stem cells and what happens to these cells in alcoholics is the first step in establishing whether the use of stem cell therapies is an option for treatment.

Summary

Alcoholics are not all alike. They experience different degrees of impairment, and the disease has different origins for different people. Consequently, researchers have not found conclusive evidence that any one variable is solely responsible for the brain deficits found in alcoholics. Characterizing what makes some alcoholics vulnerable to brain damage whereas others are not remains the subject of active research.

The good news is that most alcoholics with cognitive impairment show at least some improvement in brain structure and functioning within a year of abstinence, though some people take much longer. Clinicians must consider a variety of treatment methods to help people stop drinking and to recover from alcohol-related brain impairments, and tailor these treatments to the individual patient.

Advanced technology will have an important role in developing these therapies. Clinicians can use brain-imaging techniques to monitor the course and success of treatment, because imaging can reveal structural, functional, and biochemical changes in living patients over time. Promising new medications also are in the early stages of development, as researchers strive to design therapies that can help prevent alcohol's harmful effects and promote the growth of new brain cells to take the place of those that have been damaged by alcohol.

Chapter 11

Alcohol And Liver Disease

Alcoholic Liver Disease

The liver is one of the largest and most complex organs in the body. It stores vital energy and nutrients; manufactures proteins and enzymes necessary for good health; protects the body from disease; and breaks down (or metabolizes) and helps remove harmful toxins, like alcohol, from the body.

Because the liver is the chief organ responsible for metabolizing alcohol, it is especially vulnerable to alcohol-related injury. Even as few as three drinks at one time may have toxic effects on the liver when combined with certain over-the-counter medications, such as those containing acetaminophen.

This chapter examines the diagnosis and treatment of alcoholic liver disease (ALD), a serious and potentially fatal consequence of drinking alcohol. Another disorder, hepatitis C, also featured here, often is found in patients with ALD.

About This Chapter: This chapter includes excerpts from "Alcohol Alert: Alcoholic Liver Disease," National Institute on Alcohol Abuse and Alcoholism (NIAAA), January 2005. Additional text under the heading "Questions And Answers About Cirrhosis Of The Liver" is from "What I Need To Know About Cirrhosis Of The Liver," National Digestive Diseases Information Clearinghouse (NDDIC), a service of the National Institute of Diabetes and Digestive and Kidney Diseases (NIDDK), October 2005.

Figure 11.1. The liver is one of the largest organs in the body. It performs many of the vital functions necessary for maintaining good health. The liver is remarkably resilient in responding to disease and infection and, in fact—under certain circumstances—can even generate whole new sections of itself to replace those that are diseased (Source: Image from NDDIC, October 2005; Information in caption from NIAAA, January 2005).

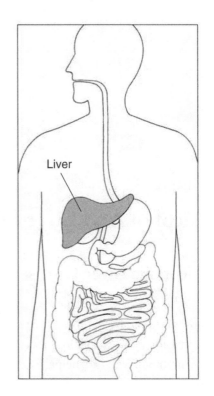

From Steatosis To Cirrhosis

Alcoholic liver disease (ALD) includes three conditions: fatty liver, alcoholic hepatitis, and cirrhosis. Heavy drinking, for as little as a few days, can lead to "fatty" liver, or steatosis—the earliest stage of alcoholic liver disease and the most common alcohol-induced liver disorder. Steatosis is marked by an excessive buildup of fat inside liver cells. This condition can be reversed, however, when drinking stops.

Drinking heavily for longer periods may lead to a more severe, and potentially fatal, condition called alcoholic hepatitis—an inflammation of the liver. Symptoms include nausea, lack of appetite, vomiting, fever, abdominal pain and tenderness, jaundice, and, sometimes, mental confusion. Scientists believe that if drinking continues (in some patients), this inflammation eventually leads to alcoholic cirrhosis, a condition where healthy liver cells are replaced by scar tissue (fibrosis), which leaves the liver unable to perform its vital functions.

Questions And Answers About Cirrhosis Of The Liver

What is cirrhosis of the liver?

Cirrhosis refers to scarring of the liver. Scar tissue forms because of injury or long-term disease. It replaces healthy tissue.

Scar tissue cannot do what healthy liver tissue does—make protein, help fight infections, clean the blood, help digest food, and store energy for when you need it. Scar tissue also blocks the normal flow of blood through the liver. Too much scar tissue means that your liver cannot work properly. To live, you need a liver that works.

Cirrhosis can be life-threatening, but it can also be controlled if treated early.

What are the symptoms of cirrhosis?

You may have no symptoms at all in the early stages. As cirrhosis progresses you may feel tired or weak, lose your appetite, feel sick to your stomach, and lose weight.

Cirrhosis can also lead to other problems.

☞ **Remember!!**

Alcohol is a toxin that is especially harmful to the liver, and alcoholic liver disease (ALD)—particularly cirrhosis—is one of the leading causes of alcohol-related death. Not everyone who drinks heavily will develop ALD. Other factors besides alcohol also influence development of the disease, including demographic, biological, and environmental factors. Nevertheless, stopping drinking can help to alleviate or even reverse ALD, especially in the early stages of disease.

Source: National Institute on Alcohol Abuse and Alcoholism (NIAAA), January 2005.

- You may bruise or bleed easily, or have nosebleeds.

- Bloating or swelling may occur as fluid builds up in the abdomen or legs. Fluid build up in the abdomen is called ascites (ah-SI-teez) and in the legs is called edema.

- Medications may have a stronger effect on you because your liver does not break them down as quickly.

- Waste materials from food may build up in the blood or brain and may cause confusion or difficulty thinking. For example, protein that you eat breaks down into chemicals like ammonia. When red blood cells get old, they break down and leave a substance called bilirubin (bil-ih-ROO-bun). A healthy liver removes these byproducts, but a diseased liver leaves them in the body.

- Blood pressure may increase in the vein entering the liver, a condition called portal hypertension.

- Enlarged veins, called varices (VARE-ah-seez), may develop in the esophagus and stomach. Varices can bleed suddenly, causing vomiting of blood or passing of blood in a bowel movement.

- The kidneys may not work properly or may fail.

- As cirrhosis progresses, your skin and the whites of your eyes may turn yellow, a condition called jaundice (JON-diss). You may also develop severe itching or gallstones.

In the early stages, cirrhosis causes your liver to swell. Then, as more scar tissue replaces normal tissue, the liver shrinks.

About five percent of patients with cirrhosis also get cancer of the liver.

What causes cirrhosis?

Cirrhosis has many causes, including those listed below.

- Alcohol abuse (alcoholic liver disease)
- Chronic viral hepatitis (hepatitis B, C, or D)

- Autoimmune hepatitis, which is the destruction of liver cells by the body's immune system

- Nonalcoholic fatty liver disease or nonalcoholic steatohepatitis (NASH), which is fat deposits and inflammation in the liver

- Some drugs, toxins, and infections

- Blocked bile ducts, the tubes that carry bile from the liver

- Some inherited diseases, including those listed below

  - Hemochromatosis, a disease that occurs when the body absorbs too much iron and stores the excess iron in the liver, pancreas, and other organs

  - Wilson disease, which is caused by the buildup of too much copper in the liver

  - Protoporphyria, a disorder that affects the skin, bone marrow, and liver

Sometimes the cause of cirrhosis remains unknown even after a thorough medical examination.

Alcoholic Hepatitis And Alcoholic Liver Disease

The presence of alcoholic hepatitis is a red flag that cirrhosis may soon follow. Up to 70 percent of all alcoholic hepatitis patients eventually develop cirrhosis. Patients with alcoholic hepatitis, who stop drinking, may have a complete recovery from liver disease, or they may still develop cirrhosis.

Liver cirrhosis is a major cause of death in the United States. In 2000, it was the 12th leading cause of death. Cirrhosis mortality rates vary substantially among age groups. They are very low among young people, but increase considerably in middle age. In fact, cirrhosis is the fourth leading cause of death in people ages 45–54.

Other factors besides alcohol may also influence ALD development, including demographic and biological factors such as ethnic and racial background,

♣ It's A Fact!!
Understanding How Alcohol Affects Your Liver

Even moderate social drinkers can experience liver damage. Diseases such as "fatty liver," hepatitis, or cirrhosis can develop from heavy alcohol consumption.

"Fatty liver" is the earliest stage of alcoholic liver disease. In this condition, liver cells become swollen with fat globules and water. If drinking is stopped at this point however, the liver is capable of healing itself.

Hepatitis is an inflammation of the liver, which causes soreness and swelling. Hepatitis can be caused by many things, such as drinking too much alcohol and taking some medications. Viruses are also a cause for hepatitis. Advanced liver damage makes it difficult for your body to break down waste products (such as bilirubin) in your blood, therefore causing jaundice, a condition where your skin turns a yellow-orange color. Waste products in the bloodstream can also cause itching, nausea, fever, and body aches.

Another serious liver disease is cirrhosis that can develop by exposure to harmful chemicals. However, the most common cause of cirrhosis in this country is drinking too much alcohol. This is better known as alcoholic cirrhosis. Alcoholic cirrhosis causes the cells of the liver to be damaged beyond repair. As liver cells die, scar tissue forms. When this scar tissue builds up, blood can't flow through the liver properly.

Normally, toxins and wastes in the blood get filtered (cleaned) out when blood passes through the liver. If scar tissue keeps blood from flowing normally through the liver, the blood doesn't get filtered. Toxins and wastes can build up in the body. This can lead to mental confusion, agitation, or tremors (shaking). In serious cases it can even lead to coma. Once scarring has progressed, nothing can be done to repair the liver or cure cirrhosis. Treatment is aimed at avoiding further damage to the liver and preventing and treating complications such as bleeding from broken blood vessels. Liver transplantation is the only option.

More than 25,000 Americans die each year from chronic liver disease. Experts say that about 70 percent are due, at least in part, to alcohol abuse. Transplants, an effective treatment for diseased livers, are not easy to come by, especially if you are currently drinking.

Source: Excerpted from "Interactive Body," National Institute on Alcohol Abuse and Alcoholism (www.collegedrinkingprevention.gov), July 11, 2007.

gender, age, education, income, employment, and a family history of drinking problems.

Women are at higher risk than men for developing cirrhosis. This higher risk may be the result of differences in the way alcohol is absorbed and broken down. When a woman drinks, the alcohol in her bloodstream reaches a higher level than in a man's bloodstream—even if both are drinking the same amount. The chemicals involved in breaking down alcohol also differ between men and women. For example, women's stomachs may contain less of a key enzyme (alcohol dehydrogenase) needed for the initial breakdown of alcohol. This means that a woman breaks down alcohol at a slower rate, exposing her liver to higher blood alcohol concentrations (BACs) for longer periods of time—a situation that is potentially toxic to the liver. Differences in how a woman's body breaks down and removes alcohol may also be linked to how much and how often she drinks, the fact that estrogen is present in her body, and even her liver size.

Diagnosing Alcoholic Liver Disease

Diagnosing alcoholic liver disease (ALD) is a challenge. A history of heavy alcohol use along with certain physical signs and positive laboratory tests for liver disease are the best indicators of disease. Alcohol dependence is not necessarily a prerequisite for ALD, and ALD can be difficult to diagnose because patients often minimize or deny their alcohol abuse. Even more confounding is the fact that physical exams and lab findings may not specifically point to ALD.

Diagnosis typically relies on laboratory tests of three liver enzymes: gamma–glutamyltransferase (GGT), aspartate aminotransferase (AST), and alanine aminotransferase (ALT). Liver disease is the most likely diagnosis if the AST level is more than twice that of ALT, a ratio some studies have found in more than 80 percent of ALD patients. An elevated level of the liver enzyme GGT is another gauge of heavy alcohol use and liver injury. Of the three enzymes, GGT is the best indicator of excessive alcohol consumption, but GGT is present in many organs and is increased by other drugs as well, so high GGT levels do not necessarily mean the patient is abusing alcohol.

♣ **It's A Fact!!**

Hepatitis C And Alcohol

Hepatitis C is a liver disease caused by the hepatitis C virus (HCV). People usually become infected after coming in contact with blood from an infected person. Sharing needles or other equipment for injecting drugs is the most common way of spreading HCV. The disease also can be spread by sexual contact. About four million people in the United States have HCV, and between 10,000 and 12,000 die each year.

HCV infection is particularly common in alcoholics with liver disease. Heavy alcohol consumption accelerates patients' progression from chronic HCV to cirrhosis (a condition in which fibrous scar tissue replaces healthy liver tissue) and liver cancer (specifically, hepatocellular carcinoma, the most common form of liver cancer). Although fewer studies have examined the effects of moderate drinking on the course of liver disease in HCV patients, there is some indication that alcohol consumption in the moderate-to-heavy range may increase HCV-infected patients' risk of developing liver fibrosis and cirrhosis. Research on whether gender has any effect on the connection between alcohol consumption and liver disease progression in HCV patients is very limited.

Treatment: Blood tests can diagnose HCV infection, either by detecting antibodies to the virus or by detecting the presence and quantity of the virus's genetic material itself. There currently is no vaccine for hepatitis C. The standard treatment includes the use of antiviral treatment (interferon-alfa with ribavirin).

Strict abstinence from alcohol is important during treatment, as heavy drinking during treatment has been shown to hinder patients' responses to therapy. In addition, depression, irritability, and anxiety—side effects that occur in 20 to 30 percent of patients who receive interferon treatment—may be especially difficult to manage in patients with a history of alcoholism, perhaps putting them at greater risk for relapsing to drinking. Thus, for treatment to be most successful, clinicians recommend that alcoholic patients abstain from drinking alcohol at least six months prior to beginning interferon therapy. Light-to-moderate drinkers can begin treatment immediately and do not need a period of abstinence before starting therapy.

Source: National Institute on Alcohol Abuse and Alcoholism (NIAAA), January 2005.

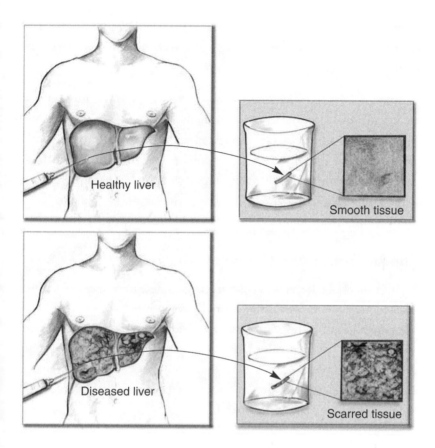

Figure 11.2. The most accurate way to diagnose cirrhosis is by liver biopsy. In a liver biopsy, a needle is used to take a small piece of liver tissue. That sample is then examined under a microscope to look for scar tissue (Source: NIDDK October 2005).

Treating Alcoholic Liver Disease

Treatment strategies for ALD include lifestyle changes to reduce alcohol consumption, cigarette smoking, and obesity; nutritional therapy; pharmacological therapy; and possibly liver transplantation (in case of cirrhosis).

Lifestyle Changes

Abstinence from alcohol is vital to prevent further liver injury, scarring, and possibly liver cancer because it appears to benefit patients at each stage of the disease. Although only a few studies have looked specifically at the effects of abstinence on the progression of ALD, virtually every one has shown that abstaining from alcohol is beneficial.

Many people who drink alcohol also smoke cigarettes, and European studies have found scarring of the liver occurs more rapidly in ALD patients who smoked. Obesity is another factor associated with liver disease—specifically, the development of fatty liver and nonalcoholic steatohepatitis, which is a disorder similar to alcoholic hepatitis. Thus, stopping smoking and maintaining a healthy weight are two more measures patients can take to reduce or prevent further liver injury.

Nutritional Treatment

Although alcoholic beverages contain calories, research suggests that under certain conditions these calories do not have as much value for the body as those derived from other nutrients. In addition, many alcoholics suffer from malnutrition, which can lead to liver damage and impaired liver function. Many drinkers take in less than the recommended daily amount of carbohydrates, proteins, fats, vitamins (A, C, and B, especially thiamine [B1]), and minerals (such as calcium and iron).

To prevent these deficiencies, clinicians should provide alcoholics with a balanced diet. Dietary supplements may prevent or relieve some of alcohol's harmful effects. For example, brain damage resulting from a lack of vitamin B1, which can lead to conditions such as Wernicke-Korsakoff syndrome, can be reversed to some extent. Because vitamin B1 generally can be administered safely, clinicians often recommend that all alcoholics undergoing treatment receive 50 milligrams of thiamine per day (either by injection if the patients are hospitalized or by mouth). Alcoholics also should receive supplements of vitamins B2 (riboflavin) and B6 (pyridoxine) in dosages found in standard multivitamins. Vitamin A, however, can be toxic when combined with alcohol and should be given only to those alcoholics who have a well-documented deficiency and who can stop or significantly reduce their drinking.

In addition to dietary supplements, alcoholics with moderate malnutrition might benefit from treatment with anabolic steroids. These compounds, which are derived from the male hormone testosterone, can be used in the short term to promote overall body "buildup" and, therefore, may help the alcoholic better recover from malnutrition.

Emerging Therapies

Studies using animals are helping researchers find other dietary supplements that may help in the treatment of liver disease. For example, eating certain healthy fats (called medium–chain triglycerides, or MCTs) may help to reduce the buildup of harmful fats in the liver. MCTs generally are available only in health food stores as a dietary supplement.

Oxidative stress plays a major role in the development of alcoholic liver disease. Oxidative stress occurs when harmful oxygen molecules, or free radicals, form in the body. These molecules are highly charged and very unstable. They cause cellular changes in their effort to pair with the nearest available molecule, injuring cells and modifying their function. Antioxidants can help prevent this free radical damage.

An important antioxidant, glutathione, or GSH, cannot be used as a supplement because this substance cannot directly enter the cells threatened by oxidative stress. However, researchers are using a precursor compound, the molecule S–adenosylmethionine (SAMe), which can enter the cells and then break down to form the helpful antioxidant. When SAMe was given to patients with alcoholic cirrhosis in a clinical trial, they were significantly less likely to die or require a liver transplant within the next two years, compared with patients who had received an inactive substance (that is, a placebo). Moreover, the study detected virtually no harmful side effects of SAMe treatment. Thus, this approach appears to hold promise for the treatment of patients with ALD.

Pharmacological Therapy

No FDA-approved therapy exists for either alcoholic cirrhosis or alcoholic hepatitis. However, several drugs have been used "off label," including pentoxifylline (PTX) and corticosteroids. PTX was shown to be effective in patients with severe alcoholic hepatitis.

Although corticosteroids are the most extensively studied form of therapy for alcoholic hepatitis, their usefulness may be only short-term. Most investigators agree that if corticosteroids are used, they should be reserved for patients with the most severe liver disease. In addition, steroids have well-documented side effects, including increasing the risk of infection, which already is substantial in patients with alcoholic hepatitis.

Transplantation

Liver transplantation currently is the only definitive treatment for severe (end stage) liver failure. A total of 41,734 liver transplants using organs from cadavers were performed in the United States between 1992 and 2001. Of these, 12.5 percent were performed in patients with ALD, and 5.8 percent were performed in patients with ALD and a concurrent infection with the

☞ **Remember!!**

Treatment for alcoholic liver disease (ALD) includes making lifestyle changes, such as stopping or decreasing alcohol use, stopping smoking, and maintaining a healthy weight. Health care providers may prescribe medications, such as pentoxifylline or prednisone, in cases of alcoholic hepatitis. And patients may want to seek nutritional supplements or complementary and alternative medicine, such as S-adenosylmethionine (SAMe) for cirrhosis. Severe ALD is best treated with transplantation in selected abstinent patients.

Source: National Institute on Alcohol Abuse and Alcoholism (NIAAA), January 2005.

hepatitis C virus (HCV), making ALD the second most frequent reason (after HCV infection alone) for transplantation.

ALD patients must undergo a thorough evaluation to determine whether they are suitable candidates for transplant. This screening addresses any co-existing medical problems, such as heart damage, cancer, pancreatitis, and osteoporosis, which might influence the outcome of the transplant. It includes a psychological evaluation to identify those patients who are most likely to remain abstinent and comply with the strict medical regimen that follows the procedure.

For transplantation to be successful in alcoholic patients it is essential that they remain abstinent after the surgery and comply with a demanding medical regimen (such as, consistently take the necessary antirejection medications). Routinely conducting psychiatric evaluations before patients are included on the list of candidates for transplantation helps to identify those who may not be able to meet these criteria.

Because of the shortage of donated organs, transplantation to patients with alcoholic liver disease remains controversial, mainly out of concern that the transplanted liver could be "wasted" if a patient relapses to drinking and damages the new liver as well. Yet the relapse rates in patients following transplant are lower than in patients undergoing alcoholism treatment, and serious relapses that adversely affect the transplanted liver or the patient are uncommon. In contrast, patients who receive a transplant because of an infection with hepatitis B or C viruses typically experience disease recurrence and are more likely to lose the transplanted liver because of recurrence of these infections.

Another concern is that patients with ALD will not be able to comply with the antirejection medication regimen, but this has not been supported by research. Liver rejection rates are similar for patients transplanted for ALD and those transplanted for other types of liver disease, indicating comparable rates of compliance with the antirejection medications. Finally, it was believed that ALD patients would use more resources, thereby incurring higher costs than non-ALD patients, but again this assumption has not been corroborated by research evidence.

In contrast to these negative assumptions on the use of liver transplants in ALD patients, many clinicians contend that ALD is, in fact, an excellent reason for liver transplantation. The overall improvement in patients with ALD after transplant, including higher productivity and better quality of life, supports considering these patients for liver transplants. Moreover, the long-term costs of transplantation and subsequent management of the alcoholic patient may well be lower than the costs of managing alcoholism and ALD without transplantation.

Chapter 12

Alcohol And The Cardiovascular System

Introduction To The Cardiovascular System

The cardiovascular system is sometimes called the blood-vascular system or simply the circulatory system. It consists of the heart, which is a muscular pumping device, and a closed system of vessels called arteries, veins, and capillaries. As the name implies, blood contained in the circulatory system is pumped by the heart around a closed circle or circuit of vessels as it passes again and again through the various "circulations" of the body.

What Is Heart Disease?

Coronary heart disease—often simply called heart disease—occurs when the arteries that supply blood to the heart muscle become hardened and narrowed due to a buildup of plaque on the arteries' inner walls. Plaque is the

About This Chapter: This chapter begins with an excerpt from the "Introduction to the Cardiovascular System," Surveillance, Epidemiology and End Results (SEER) Program, National Cancer Institute, 2000. "What Is Heart Disease?" is excerpted from "Your Guide to a Healthy Heart," National Heart, Lung, and Blood Institute, NIH Pub. No. 06-5269, November 2005. Excerpts from "Alcohol's Effects On The Risk For Coronary Heart Disease," by Kenneth J. Mukamal, M.D., M.P.H., M.A., and Eric B. Rimm, Sc.D, National Institute on Alcohol Abuse and Alcoholism (NIAAA), 2001, are also included. The full text of this document, including references, can be found online at http://pubs.niaaa.nih.gov/publications/arh25-4/255-261.pdf. The information in this chapter was reviewed for currency by David A. Cooke, M.D., in December 2008.

accumulation of fat, cholesterol, and other substances. As plaque continues to build up in the arteries, blood flow to the heart is reduced.

Heart disease can lead to a heart attack. A heart attack happens when an artery becomes totally blocked with plaque, preventing vital oxygen and nutrients from getting to the heart. A heart attack can cause permanent damage to the heart muscle. Heart disease is one of several cardiovascular diseases, which are disorders of the heart and blood vessel system. Other cardiovascular diseases include stroke, high blood pressure, and rheumatic heart disease.

Some people aren't too concerned about heart disease because they think it can be "cured" with surgery. This is a myth. Heart disease is a lifelong condition: Once you get it, you'll always have it. It's true that procedures such as angioplasty and bypass surgery can help blood and oxygen flow more easily to the heart. But the arteries remain damaged, which means you are still more likely to have a heart attack. What's more, the condition of your blood vessels will steadily worsen unless you make changes in your daily habits and control your risk factors. Many people die of complications from heart disease, or become permanently disabled. That's why it is so vital to take action to prevent this disease.

Alcohol's Effects On The Risk For Coronary Heart Disease

Several studies have indicated that moderate drinkers have a lower risk of both nonfatal myocardial infarction and fatal heart disease than do abstainers. Since the early part of the 20th century, clinicians have noted that coronary heart disease appears to occur less commonly among people who consume alcohol than among abstainers. Over the last 30 years, formal scientific inquiry has confirmed this observation. Such analyses included studies that compared alcohol use between people with and without confirmed coronary disease (that is, case-control studies) as well as studies that followed healthy drinkers and abstainers over time to determine their risk of coronary disease (that is, prospective cohort studies). Both types of studies found that people who consumed alcohol in moderation had lower rates of coronary heart disease compared with abstainers. Similarly, the drinkers had a 16 percent lower risk of undergoing bypass surgery or angioplasty compared with abstainers. These findings were confirmed in a review of over 50 epidemiological studies, which concluded that compared to total abstinence, consumption of one drink every one to two days is associated with a 17 percent lower risk of nonfatal myocardial infarction.

♣ It's A Fact!!
Heavy Drinking And Heart Disease

Heavy drinking causes many heart-related problems. More than three drinks per day can raise blood pressure and triglyceride levels, while binge drinking can contribute to stroke. Too much alcohol also can damage the heart muscle, leading to heart failure. Overall, people who drink heavily on a regular basis have higher rates of heart disease than either moderate drinkers or nondrinkers.

Source: National Heart, Lung, and Blood Institute, NIH
Pub. No. 06-5269, November 2005.

Does Alcohol Truly Prevent Coronary Heart Disease?

Although the evidence of a lower risk of coronary heart disease among moderate drinkers is substantial and consistent, controversy remains about whether the relationship is truly causal—that is, whether moderate alcohol consumption really prevents coronary heart disease. For example, some investigators have argued that abstainers are an inappropriate control population because at least some of these people may abstain because of illness or former alcohol abuse. Furthermore, other dietary, lifestyle, and developmental factors may differ between abstainers and drinkers. Both of these concerns warrant closer scrutiny.

The first of these concerns, also called the "sick quitter" hypothesis, was proposed by researchers in the United Kingdom. It states that the pool of abstainers includes many former drinkers who quit drinking because of illness or because alcohol interacts with prescription drugs they are taking.

Obviously, comparisons of healthy drinkers with abstainers who take prescription drugs or who have underlying illnesses that raise one's risk for heart disease will produce a biased result in favor of the alcohol-consuming subjects.

Similarly, alcoholic patients in recovery rarely return to moderate, or social, drinking. Thus, people who have alcoholism—whether still active or in remission—will tend toward the extremes of alcohol consumption. People with active alcoholism, however, tend to be under-represented in large, prospective studies of heart disease. As a result, comparison of drinkers (who under-represent active alcohol abusers) to abstainers (who include recovering alcoholics) may produce misleading results if heavy alcohol consumption contributes to a higher risk of heart disease. A similar bias may occur if, in self-report surveys, people who consume alcohol in excess deliberately describe themselves as abstainers because of the social stigma attached to alcohol abuse.

Other fundamental differences also exist between abstainers and drinkers. For example, abstainers tend to come from less welcoming childhood environments and to report poorer health than do drinkers, even in early adulthood. Moreover, many abstainers have chosen to forsake alcohol intake because of adverse experiences with alcoholic family members. Such differences, which might influence a person's underlying risk of heart disease, are difficult to account for with standard epidemiological or statistical methods.

> ## ♣ It's A Fact!!
> Some people should not drink at all.
>
> - Anyone under age 21
> - People of any age who are unable to restrict their drinking to moderate levels
> - Women who may become pregnant or who are pregnant
> - People who plan to drive, operate machinery, or take part in other activities that require attention, skill, or coordination
> - People taking prescription or over-the-counter medications that can interact with alcohol
>
> Source: "Alcohol: A Women's Health Issue," National Institute on Alcohol Abuse and Alcoholism (NIAAA), March 2005.

Finally, the level of alcohol consumption is a marker for several lifestyle factors that strongly influence health. Moderate drinkers tend to be younger, leaner, more physical active, of higher socioeconomic status, and more likely to be married compared with people who abstain or drink rarely. All of these factors have been shown to influence one's risk of coronary heart disease.

Approaches For Accounting For Potential Confounding Factors

Researchers have sought to address these concerns in several ways. Some epidemiological studies have separated former drinkers from long-term abstainers to address the sick quitter hypothesis. For example, in an analysis of 87,526 women, the risk of coronary heart disease was only 10 percent higher among former drinkers than among long-term abstainers. Furthermore, the exclusion of former drinkers among the abstainers did not alter the 40 percent lower risk of coronary heart disease among women who drank 5.0 to 14.9 grams of alcohol (about 0.3 to one standard drink) daily. Moreover, researchers found comparable risks of coronary heart disease among abstainers and light drinkers (that is, people who consumed less than 5.0 grams of alcohol, or 0.3 standard drinks, daily) in their study of 51,529 healthy men, suggesting that abstainers are not an inappropriate reference group. Other studies have excluded participants who developed coronary heart disease or died during the first few years of follow-up, as a means of excluding unidentified "sick" subjects, with similar results. Taken together these findings indicate that the presence of sick quitters or former alcoholics among the abstainers is not responsible for the apparent benefits of alcohol consumption on the risk of coronary heart disease.

Researchers also have sought to separate the confounding influence of dietary, lifestyle, and socioeconomic factors from the role of alcohol consumption itself. In the separate prospective studies of men and women noted earlier, researchers controlled for the participants' body-mass index (a measure of obesity) and dietary intake of cholesterol, saturated fat, and polyunsaturated fat. These analyses confirmed that diet alone is unlikely to have caused the apparent effect of alcohol consumption on heart disease. Studies that have controlled for the participants' social integration, social class, physical activity, or occupation have reported similar results.

> **♣ It's A Fact!!**
>
> One area of controversy remains the role of the type of beverage a drinker consumes preferentially. The French paradox—the observation that the rate of coronary heart disease in France is relatively low despite high rates of saturated fat intake and cigarette smoking—has led to the belief that red wine is particularly beneficial for health. This specific effect has been suggested to result from the antioxidant properties of some components of red wine rather than its alcohol content. However, observational studies have not consistently shown a difference in the risk of heart disease between wine drinkers and consumers of other alcoholic beverages.
>
> Source: Mukaml, et. al., NIAAA, 2001.

In summary, all of this evidence implicates alcohol consumption rather than lifestyle factors (including those that correlate with the consumption of specific beverage types) as the primary factor in the lower rates of cardiovascular disease found among moderate drinkers.

Approaches To Defining The Causal Role Of Alcohol

Although investigators have used a variety of approaches to address the aforementioned concerns, the most definitive way to determine whether alcohol consumption itself prevents coronary heart disease would be to conduct a randomized trial. Because the participants are randomly assigned to the active or control treatment and all participants are equally likely to receive a given treatment, the design of a randomized trial minimizes the effects of other variables. For an agent such as alcohol, which is influenced by, and in turn influences, so many other factors, the advantages of a randomized study design are particularly useful.

Unfortunately, however, even the randomized trial is not a perfect tool for determining the relationship between alcohol consumption and coronary heart disease. No long-term trial of alcohol administration has ever been performed, nor is one likely in the near future. Such a trial would face substantial hurdles.

- High costs

- An inability to prevent participants from knowing whether they receive alcohol

- The need to find large numbers of people who are not prevented from using alcohol for medical reasons and who are willing to forgo or continue alcohol use for long periods of time

- The possibility that some participants instructed to consume alcohol would eventually misuse it or even become alcohol dependent

In contrast, researchers have conducted many randomized short-term trials of alcohol administration and its consequences. These trials avoid the pitfalls of observational studies (for example, the influences of factors that cannot easily be measured) and the concerns associated with long-term trials. The interpretability of such short-term studies, however, often is limited. For example, short-term trials of alcohol use are necessarily limited to studying physiological measures (for example, changes in blood cholesterol levels) rather than clinical endpoints (for example, the development of heart disease). The relevance of such physiological measures to clinical heart disease, however, is often uncertain. Furthermore, because they often include small numbers of subjects, these trials produce relatively imprecise results.

Alcohol's Effects On Coronary Risk Factors

As mentioned previously, the findings of observational studies had suggested that alcohol consumption was inversely related to myocardial infarction. These findings were confirmed by the meta-analysis of short-term trials of alcohol administration, which indicated that alcohol consumption has important effects on factors involved in atherosclerosis, inflammation, and thrombosis. The most important of these effects is on high-density lipoprotein cholesterol (HDL-C, "good" cholesterol) levels. Thus, in their meta-analysis, researchers estimated that consumption of 30 grams of alcohol, or approximately two standard drinks, per day increases HDL-C levels by 4.0 milligrams per deciliter (mg/dL). This increase in HDL-C levels is greater than that produced by gemfibrozil, a medication used to treat people with low HDL-C levels and translates into a 16.8 percent decrease in the risk of coronary heart disease.

At the same time, however, alcohol consumption raises the levels of another type of fat in the blood—the triglycerides, which are associated with an increased risk of coronary heart disease. In the randomized trials included in the meta-analysis, consumption of 30 grams of alcohol raised triglyceride levels by an estimated 5.7 percent, which translates into a 4.6 percent increase in coronary heart disease. Thus, alcohol has a mixed effect on coronary risk factors by increasing both HDL-C and triglyceride levels. The balance of these effects, however, appears to favor prevention of coronary heart disease.

✤ It's A Fact!!
Alcohol: Cardiac Risks As Well As Benefits

The heart has the important job of getting oxygen to every cell in the body. Accomplishing this task is not that easy for such a small organ, as it weighs between 7 and 15 ounces.

Some research has indicated that having some alcohol can provide health benefits to the heart. However, drinking alcohol, even in moderation, can create health risks such as a slight rise in blood pressure. High blood pressure associated with heavy drinking makes the heart work harder than it needs to and can be a key risk factor for coronary heart disease, leading to heart attacks and strokes. In addition, with increased intake of alcohol, levels of some fats in the blood can become elevated (high blood triglycerides), which could cause heart problems.

Excessive drinking of alcohol (binge drinking) can also lead to stroke and other serious health problems. These other problems can include cardiomyopathy (disease of the heart muscle), cardiac arrhythmia (abnormal contraction patterns of the heart) and sudden cardiac death.

Source: Excerpted from "Interactive Body," National Institute on Alcohol Abuse and Alcoholism (www.collegedrinkingprevention.gov), July 11, 2007.

The meta-analysis also detected important effects of alcohol consumption on blood-clotting (that is, coagulatory) factors. The best studied of these factors is fibrinogen, which is converted to fibrin during blood clot formation. The randomized short-term trials of alcohol administration included in the meta-analysis indicated that consumption of 30 grams of alcohol lowered fibrinogen levels by an estimated 7.5 mg/dL. This degree of reduction in fibrinogen concentration would be expected to reduce the risk of heart disease by 12.5 percent.

Taken together, the estimated changes in HDL-C, triglyceride, and fibrinogen levels induced by consumption of 30 grams of alcohol appear to result in a 24.7 percent reduction in the risk of coronary heart disease. Thus, the results of the randomized trials included in that meta-analysis support the hypothesis that alcohol indeed is the cause of the lower rates of coronary heart disease found among moderate drinkers, although additional research is needed to prove this assumption.

Other Potential Mechanisms Of Alcohol's Effects

Alcohol consumption may also affect the risk of coronary heart disease by acting on other proteins involved in blood clot formation and fibrinolysis, as well as on platelet aggregation, blood pressure, and inflammation. For example, the meta-analysis researchers found that consumption of 30 grams of alcohol raises the levels of the fibrinolytic protein tissue-type plasminogen activator (t-PA) by approximately 20 percent. Such an increase in t-PA levels might be expected to lower the risk of coronary heart disease; however, observational studies found the opposite effect (that is, an increased risk of heart disease). One explanation for this observation might be that higher t-PA concentrations generally reflect more extensive underlying vascular disease. Alternatively, much of the measured t-PA in the blood may be bound to its inhibitor, plasminogen activator inhibitor-1, and therefore be inactive.

Furthermore, the meta-analysis found that intake of 30 grams of alcohol is associated with a 0.70 mg/dL decrease in the levels of a molecule called Lp (a) lipoprotein, which is a lipid particle that may influence fibrinolytic activity. The relationship between Lp (a) lipoprotein and the risk of vascular disease has been inconsistent, however.

Alcohol also appears to inhibit platelet aggregation. This observation was confirmed in the randomized experimental studies included in the meta-analysis, which used a variety of tests. These studies found generally consistent evidence that alcohol consumption prevents platelet aggregation.

Although the relevance of these findings for the risk for coronary heart disease is less clear than with confirmed coronary risk factors, such as HDL-C or fibrinogen, alcohol's effects on platelet activity could represent an important mechanism through which alcohol could prevent cardiovascular disease.

Alcohol intake may also affect the inflammation associated with atherosclerotic plaques and the function of the cells that line the blood vessels (that is, endothelial cells). Observational studies indicate that moderate drinkers have lower levels of markers of inflammation. These markers include a molecule called C-reactive protein that is produced during inflammatory states and which has been linked to increased risk of coronary heart disease. Conversely observational studies also indicate that moderate drinkers have higher levels of homocysteine, a substance derived from breakdown of the amino acid methionine that may increase the risk of blood clots. Only modest experimental data exist, however, to confirm either relationship.

> ♣ **It's A Fact!!**
> Alcohol appears to have important effects on cardiovascular risk factors. Among the most controversial of these risk factors is blood pressure. Both epidemiological evidence and clinical trials confirm that heavy drinking (that is, three or more standard drinks per day) raises blood pressure, both among people with and without elevated blood pressure (that is, hypertension) prior to alcohol consumption. However, the effects of smaller amounts of alcohol on blood pressure have not been widely tested in randomized trials, and observational studies do not support a substantial effect on blood pressure from moderate drinking.
>
> Source: Mukaml, et. al. NIAAA, 2001.

Small studies have found mixed results of the effect of alcohol consumption on the function of the endothelial lining of the blood vessels. Laboratory experiments have suggested that regular alcohol consumption might increase the endothelial cells' production of and responsiveness to nitric oxide, a small molecule made in blood vessel walls that helps to relax constricted blood vessels and thereby improve blood flow to organs such as the heart. If these findings can be confirmed, they could suggest another mechanism through which alcohol consumption may prevent myocardial infarction.

The Role Of Genetic Factors In The Association Of Alcohol And Heart Disease

One unresolved question is whether the relationship of alcohol consumption to heart disease is consistent throughout the general population or differs among certain subgroups (for example, men and women). Because men and women differ in how they metabolize alcohol and in their under-lying risk of cardiovascular disease, for example, they may also differ in how alcohol consumption relates to their risk of heart disease. Such variability is difficult to assess in randomized trials of alcohol consumption, which have been too small to allow subgroup comparisons. Observational studies, however, provide some intriguing answers to this question. For example, the studies of healthy men and women, mentioned previously, suggest that moderate drinking is associated with lower risk of heart disease in both sexes, despite the differences in alcohol metabolism and risk of cardiovascular disease. These studies also demonstrate, however, that the level of alcohol consumption associated with the lowest risk of heart disease is lower among women than among men, consistent with public health recommendations that advise consumption of no more than two drinks per day for men and no more than one drink per day for nonpregnant women.

Genetic factors may also modify the relationship between moderate drinking and coronary heart disease in interesting ways. For example, the initial breakdown of the alcohol contained in alcoholic beverages—chemically referred to as ethanol—is mediated by an enzyme called alcohol dehydrogenase (ADH). Three different versions of ADH exist—ADH1, ADH2, and ADH3. Of these, ADH3 has two common genetic variants, or alleles, that break down ethanol at different speeds (that is, fast and slow). Each person carries two copies of the ADH3 gene, one inherited from the father and one inherited from the mother. Accordingly, a person can carry either two fast alleles, two slow alleles, or one fast and one slow allele of the ADH3 gene.

A recent study of 396 men with myocardial infarction and 770 control men studied the relationship between these ADH3 alleles and the risk of heart disease. The study found that compared with men who carried two copies of the fast allele and drank less than once per week, men who carried two copies of the fast allele (and drank daily) had a 38 percent lower risk of myocardial infarction. In contrast, daily drinkers who had two copies of the slow allele had an 86 percent lower risk of myocardial infarction compared with men with two slow alleles (who drank less than weekly). These results suggest that, within the range of moderate drinking, greater exposure time to alcohol (on the basis of more frequent drinking and slower metabolism) may lower one's risk of myocardial infarction.

♣ **It's A Fact!!**
Once thought of as a threat mainly to men, heart disease also is the leading killer of women in the United States. Drinking moderately may lower the risk for coronary heart disease, mainly among women over age 55. However, there are other factors that reduce the risk of heart disease, including a healthy diet, exercise, not smoking, and keeping a healthy weight. Moderate drinking provides little, if any, net health benefit for younger people, and heavy drinking can actually damage the heart.

Source: "Alcohol: A Women's Health Issue," National Institute on Alcohol Abuse and Alcoholism (NIAAA), January 2005.

The researchers also found that among daily drinkers, "good" HDL-C cholesterol increased with the number of slow ADH3 alleles—that is, daily drinkers with two slow ADH3 alleles had higher HDL-C levels than did daily drinkers with no slow ADH3 allele levels; men with one slow allele had intermediate HDL-C levels. This finding provides a plausible explanation for the gene-related variation in the relationship between alcohol consumption and risk of myocardial infarction described in the study.

Danish investigators reported intriguing findings in a study of 3,383 men. The investigators compared the risk of cardiovascular mortality among men with different Lewis blood group types. Much like the common ABO blood group system, a person's Lewis blood type can include just an "a" component (a+b-), just a "b" component (a-b+), both components (a+b+), or neither component (a-b-). People with the a-b- blood type seem to be at higher risk for diabetes and cardiovascular mortality than people with other Lewis blood types. In the study, men with Lewis blood group type a-b- who consumed 22 or more drinks per week had an 80 percent lower risk of coronary heart disease than did men who consumed zero to 10 drinks per week. Among men with other Lewis blood group types, however, alcohol consumption was not appreciably related to the risk of heart disease.

Taken together, these two studies suggest that genetic factors that influence potentially beneficial variables linked to alcohol use (for example, HDL-C levels) or the baseline risk of heart disease (for example, Lewis blood type groups) may modify the link between alcohol consumption and heart disease in important and informative ways.

Putting It Together

This chapter has explored whether alcohol consumption per se is responsible for the lower risk of coronary heart disease among moderate drinkers. Based on the results of the meta-analysis of randomized trials by researchers, the answer appears to be yes. If alcohol consumption indeed influences HDL-C, triglyceride, and fibrinogen levels to the degree documented in the meta-analysis, consumption of two standard drinks daily would be expected to lower a person's risk of coronary heart disease by nearly 25 percent, a figure that agrees well with the results of observational studies.

♣ It's A Fact!!

If you don't drink, the American Heart Association advises against starting to drink to reduce the risk of heart disease. The best methods for preventing heart disease are exercise, healthy diet, and avoiding all forms of tobacco exposure.

Source: Excerpted from "Alcoholism," © 2007 A.D.A.M., Inc. Reprinted with permission.

Obviously, however, alcohol consumption also has serious and important health effects other than those related to coronary heart disease. Achieving a balance between the health risks and benefits of alcohol consumption remains difficult, as each person has a different susceptibility to the adverse health consequences associated with alcohol consumption. Because each person has a unique combination of factors—such as age, sex, and family history—that influence that person's risk of specific diseases potentially caused or prevented by alcohol use, the balance of the risks and benefits of alcohol consumption for each person likewise will be unique. Accordingly, a young woman with a family history of alcoholism should weigh the decision of how much alcohol to drink (if any) differently than should a middle-aged man with a family history of premature heart disease.

☞ Remember!!

In light of the substantial and often contradictory evidence regarding the health effects of alcohol consumption, one cannot make a simple recommendation regarding the "optimal" level of alcohol consumption. In the absence of such a straightforward recommendation, adults should consult their physicians regarding the safety or risk of alcohol consumption and make personalized decisions accordingly.

Source: Mukaml, et. al. NIAAA, 2001.

One approach to examining the combined results of potentially detrimental and beneficial effects associated with alcohol consumption is to assess the overall rates of death in people who consume different amounts of alcohol. Such studies of all-cause mortality can combine the baseline risk of dying from each specific disease with the increase or decrease in the risk for that disease associated with alcohol consumption. Obviously, observational studies of all-cause mortality are susceptible to the same concerns discussed earlier regarding studies of coronary heart disease. Nevertheless, the apparent agreement of clinical and observational studies regarding the relationship between alcohol consumption and coronary heart disease provides reassurance about the validity of these reports.

Given that over 30 percent of deaths in the United States are attributable to heart disease, making it the nation's leading cause of death, it is not surprising that observational studies show that moderate drinkers have lower overall death rates than do abstainers or heavy drinkers. For example, in an American Cancer Society study of 490,000 adults, death rates among middle-aged and elderly men and women were lowest among people who consumed approximately one drink per day. In fact, death rates among these moderate drinkers were approximately 20 percent lower than among abstainers. The level of alcohol consumption associated with the lowest overall death rate, however, differed substantially based on the participants' age and risk of heart disease. For example, among participants aged 30–59 years and free of hypertension, diabetes, or cardiovascular disease, the lowest death rate was found with a consumption of less than one drink daily. Conversely, among participants aged 60–79 years and with one of these conditions, the lowest death rate occurred with a consumption of three drinks per day.

Chapter 13

Alcohol And The Digestive System

Mouth And Esophagus

The first things alcohol comes in contact with, when consumed, are the oral cavity, pharynx, and esophagus. Because the alcohol is in an undiluted state, mucosal lesions are quite common. The amount of alcohol to do this varies from person to person and depends on other factors—such as, is the stomach full or empty. That said, it is known that the risk for tissue damage goes up when over four drinks (two ounces alcohol) are consumed.

Inflammation of the tongue (that is, glossitis), the mouth (that is, stomatitis) may occur either from alcohol consumption damaging the salivary glands or poor nutrition that oftentimes goes along with heavy alcohol misuse. Other effects on the mouth can be seen in an increased incidence of tooth decay, gum disease, and tooth loss.

Heavy alcohol consumption—more than 21 standard drinks in one week—is the second largest risk factor for oral cancer. Alcohol dehydrates the cell walls, and, for smokers, increases the absorption of tobacco carcinogens through the mouth tissues. Deficiencies in nutrients associated with heavy

About This Chapter: This chapter includes information by S. Rennie, LPN, from "Mouth And Esophagus," "Stomach," "Small Intestine," and "Large Intestine," © 2008 National Alliance of Advocates for Buprenorphine Treatment. Reprinted with permission. To view the complete texts, including references, visit www.alcoholanswers.org.

♣ It's A Fact!!
Your Digestive System And How It Works

The digestive system is made up of the digestive tract—a series of hollow organs joined in a long, twisting tube from the mouth to the anus—and other organs that help the body break down and absorb food.

Organs that make up the digestive tract are the mouth, esophagus, stomach, small intestine, large intestine—also called the colon—rectum, and anus. Inside these hollow organs is a lining called the mucosa. In the mouth, stomach, and small intestine, the mucosa contains tiny glands that produce juices to help digest food. The digestive tract also contains a layer of smooth muscle that helps break down food and move it along the tract.

Two "solid" digestive organs, the liver and the pancreas, produce digestive juices that reach the intestine through small tubes called ducts. The gallbladder stores the liver's digestive juices until they are needed in the intestine. Parts of the nervous and circulatory systems also play major roles in the digestive system.

Why is digestion important?

When you eat foods—such as bread, meat, and vegetables—they are not in a form that the body can use as nourishment. Food and drink must be changed into smaller molecules of nutrients before they can be absorbed into the blood and carried to cells throughout the body. Digestion is the process by which food and drink are broken down into their smallest parts so the body can use them to build and nourish cells and to provide energy.

How is food digested?

Digestion involves mixing food with digestive juices, moving it through the digestive tract, and breaking down large molecules of food into smaller molecules. Digestion begins in the mouth, when you chew and swallow, and is completed in the small intestine.

Source: "Your Digestive System And How It Works," National Digestive Diseases Information Clearinghouse (NDDIC), a service of the National Institute of Diabetes and Digestive and Kidney Diseases (NIDDK), April 2008.

alcohol consumption can lower the ability to utilize antioxidants to prevent cancerous formations.

The esophagus, which leads to the stomach, can be damaged by even one acute alcohol consumption episode. Gastroesophageal reflux can occur due to the weakening of the lower esophageal sphincter. This, in turn, can lower the ability of the esophagus to clear the refluxed gastric acid, thus causing heartburn. "Nutcracker esophagus," an esophageal motility that has symptoms similar to coronary heart disease, can also occur in some alcohol-dependent persons.

Other esophageal maladies which may occur are: Barrett esophagus, which occurs in 10 to 20 percent of those suffering with symptomatic gastroesophageal

♣ It's A Fact!!
The Esophagus

The esophagus carries food and liquids from the mouth to the stomach. The stomach slowly pumps the food and liquids into the intestine, which then absorbs needed nutrients. This process is automatic and people are usually not aware of it. People sometimes feel their esophagus when they swallow something too large, try to eat too quickly, or drink very hot or cold liquids.

The muscular layers of the esophagus are normally pinched together at both the upper and lower ends by muscles called sphincters. When a person swallows, the sphincters relax to allow food or drink to pass from the mouth into the stomach. The muscles then close rapidly to prevent the food or drink from leaking out of the stomach back into the esophagus and mouth.

Source: "Barrett's Esophagus," National Digestive Diseases Information Clearinghouse (NDDIC), a service of the National Institute of Diabetes and Digestive and Kidney Diseases (NIDDK), July 2008.

reflux disease. This condition is characterized by changes in the cell layer lining of the esophagus, which causes abnormal acid production. Barrett esophagus can put patients at an increased risk of cancer of the esophagus because the altered cells can become cancerous.

♣ It's A Fact!!

Barrett Esophagus And Gastroesophageal Reflux Disease (GERD)

What is Barrett esophagus?

Barrett esophagus is a condition in which the tissue lining the esophagus—the muscular tube that connects the mouth to the stomach—is replaced by tissue that is similar to the lining of the intestine. This process is called intestinal metaplasia.

No signs or symptoms are associated with Barrett esophagus, but it is commonly found in people with gastroesophageal reflux disease (GERD). A small number of people with Barrett esophagus develop a rare but often deadly type of cancer of the esophagus.

Barrett esophagus affects about one percent of adults in the United States. The average age at diagnosis is 50, but determining when the problem started is usually difficult. Men develop Barrett esophagus twice as often as women, and Caucasian men are affected more frequently than men of other races. Barrett esophagus is uncommon in children.

What is gastroesophageal reflux disease (GERD)?

GERD is a more serious form of gastroesophageal reflux (GER). GER occurs when the lower esophageal sphincter opens spontaneously for varying periods of time or does not close properly and stomach contents rise into the esophagus. GER is also called acid reflux or acid regurgitation because digestive juices called acids rise with the food or fluid.

When GER occurs, food or fluid can be tasted in the back of the mouth. When refluxed stomach acid touches the lining of the esophagus it may cause

Mallory-Weiss syndrome is massive bleeding caused by tears in the mucosa at the base of the esophagus leading to the stomach. For 20 to 50 percent of patients, this comes from increased gastric pressure from repeated retching and vomiting after heavy alcohol consumption.

---

a burning sensation in the chest or throat called heartburn or acid indigestion. Occasional GER is common and does not necessarily mean one has GERD.

Persistent reflux that occurs more than twice a week is considered GERD and can eventually lead to more serious health problems. Overall, 10 to 20 percent of Americans experience GERD symptoms every day, making it one of the most common medical conditions. People of all ages can have GERD.

People who have GERD symptoms should consult with a physician. If GERD is left untreated over a long period of time, it can lead to complications such as a bleeding ulcer. Scars from tissue damage can lead to strictures—narrowed areas of the esophagus—that make swallowing difficult. GERD may also cause hoarseness, chronic cough, and conditions such as asthma.

Gastroesophageal Reflux Disease (GERD) And Barrett Esophagus

The exact causes of Barrett esophagus are not known, but GERD is a risk factor for the condition. Although people who do not have GERD can have Barrett esophagus, the condition is found about three to five times more often in people who also have GERD.

Since Barrett esophagus is more commonly seen in people with GERD, most physicians recommend treating GERD symptoms with acid-reducing drugs.

Improvement in GERD symptoms may lower the risk of developing Barrett esophagus. A surgical procedure may be recommended if medications are not effective in treating GERD.

Source: "Barrett's Esophagus," National Digestive Diseases Information Clearinghouse (NDDIC), a service of the National Institute of Diabetes and Digestive and Kidney Diseases (NIDDK), July 2008.

Stomach

Alcohol, even in relatively small amounts, can interfere with many stomach functions such as, altered gastric acid secretion, acute gastric mucosal injury, and interference with gastric and intestinal motility.

Gastric acid and digestive enzymes help break food down in the stomach. The production of excessive gastric acid may irritate the mucosa thus causing pain and could result in ulcers. In a study, it was found that alcoholic beverages such as beer and wine—with a low alcohol content—greatly increase the secretion of gastric acid and the gastric hormone gastrin, and then induces acid secretion. On the other hand, high-alcohol content beverages

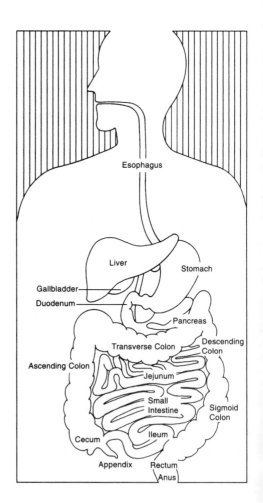

Figure 13.1. The organs of the digestive system.

> **✎ What's It Mean?**
>
> Motility: Biology. Moving or capable of moving spontaneously: motile cells; motile spores.
>
> Source: © 2008 National Alliance of Advocates for Buprenorphine Treatment.

The stomach is designed to process and transport food. Ingesting healthy foods makes this organ run smoothly.

After ingestion, alcohol travels down the esophagus into the stomach, where some of it is absorbed into your bloodstream. The unabsorbed alcohol continues to move through the gastrointestinal tract. The majority of it will enter the small intestine and get absorbed into the bloodstream through the walls of the small intestine, or it can stay in the stomach and cause irritation.

While in the stomach, alcohol acts as an irritant and increases digestive juices (hydrochloric acid) that are secreted from the stomach lining. Intoxicating amounts of alcohol can halt the digestive process, robbing the body of vital vitamins and minerals. Chronic irritation may lead to damage to the lining of the stomach.

Drinking alcohol and taking medication that causes stomach irritation, such as aspirin, can cause gastritis (inflammation of the stomach lining), ulcers, and severe bleeding.

Source: Excerpted from "Interactive Body," National Institute on Alcohol Abuse and Alcoholism (www.collegedrinkingprevention.gov), July 11, 2007.

such as whisky and cognac do not increase gastric acid secretion or the release of gastrin. The reasons for this have not yet been found. Alcohol may topically stimulate the gastric mucosa or it may be more general—affecting hormone release and regulating nerve functions connected to acid secretion. Additionally, it has been found that by-products of the fermentation of beer stimulate gastric acid secretion, and not the alcohol.

Chronic alcohol consumption can shrink the gastric mucosa and decrease gastric secretion. This lower gastric acid production inhibits the stomach's ability to kill food-related bacteria thus causing potentially harmful microorganisms to populate the upper small intestine. This can be partially reversed by abstinence.

Although it is not known how alcohol damages the gastric mucosa, it is known that alcohol consumption can cause inflammation of the mucosa and is a major cause of bleeding gastric lesions. Parts of the mucosa can be damaged or destroyed by the bleeding lesions. This generally does not happen with low to moderate alcohol consumption in a healthy person. It is more likely to happen from even just one episode of heavy drinking.

More damage that can occur during just one heavy drinking episode is the weakening of the lower esophageal sphincter. This is the two bands of muscle fibers at the end of the esophagus and the beginning of the stomach. Weakening this sphincter can cause gastroesophageal reflux. Gastroesophageal reflux can lead to heartburn, inflammation and ulcers in that part of the esophagus. This also can be damaged during one single heavy drinking episode.

Other muscle functions with which alcohol can interfere are those around the stomach wall and small intestine. This affects the time to move food through both organs. Beverages, with alcohol contents 15 percent or more, appear to delay the movement of food through the stomach. This could result in bacteria causing gases that, in turn, could cause feelings of being full and stomach discomfort.

One important piece of information to take away from this topic is that while chronic alcohol dependence and alcohol abuse cause many stomach problems, even one single heavy drinking episode can cause much damage.

Small Intestine

The small intestine is the connection between the stomach and the large intestine. About 20 feet long, it is divided into three sections: the duodenum, the jejunum and ileum. The intestinal glands secrete juices that help with digestion, and the primary purpose is to convert partially digested food into energy. Most nutrients from digested food get absorbed from the intestines into the blood and then brought to the liver.

Poor nutrition and intestines damaged by alcohol can lead to nutrient absorption difficulties. As an example, cells lining the small intestine can be altered from a lack of folate. This then hinders absorption of water, sodium, glucose, some amino acids, and fatty acids in the jejunum and ileum. Carbohydrate, protein, and fat absorption are decreased in the duodenum.

Many enzyme activities needed for proper functioning of the intestines can be disrupted by alcohol consumption. Lactase, for one, is an enzyme that breaks down lactose. A deficiency in lactase can cause lactose intolerance.

These enzymes that help transport nutrients from the intestine to the bloodstream can be compromised by alcohol consumption. It can also inhibit the enzymes that work in the metabolizing of drugs and foreign organic substances.

A single episode of heavy alcohol consumption could cause erosions and bleeding in the upper part of the duodenum. This is caused by different reactions: 1) The alcohol, itself, doing the damage. 2) The release of noxious signaling molecules (that is, cytokines, histamine, and leukotrienes), which alcohol signals. Lesions caused by either of these allow large molecules (that is, endotoxins and other bacterial toxins) to enter the bloodstream and lymph. These molecules can then enter the bloodstream, reach the liver, and possibly cause damage to it. One more causal effect is the resulting changes in capillaries that lead to mucosal injuries.

One last effect is on the muscle movements that help keep food in the small intestine for further digestion. These movements can be slowed by alcohol, resulting in heightened sensitivity to foods with high sugar contents and faster food movement through the intestines, resulting in diarrhea.

Large Intestine

The large intestine is almost five feet long and divided into six parts: cecum, ascending colon, transverse colon, descending colon, sigmoid colon, and the rectum. Partially digested food enters the large intestine from the small intestine via the ileocecal valve. The main purpose of the large intestine is to digest food further, release nutrients into the bloodstream, and absorb fluids.

Alcohol consumption greatly reduces the frequency and strength of muscle contractions in the rectum. This, as in the small intestine, can speed movement of food through the intestines thus reducing absorption of nutrients and fluids and also cause diarrhea.

Epidemiological human data and biochemical animal experimental data both show that chronic alcohol consumption poses a great risk factor for polyps and cancer of the colorectum. This can occur as alcohol may act as a cocarcinogen by enhancing the carcinogen effects of other chemicals and also interacting with enzymes that normally help detoxify substances in the body. This interaction can also increase the toxicity of some carcinogens, which results in cancer.

Chapter 14

Alcohol And The Pancreas

Pancreatitis

What is pancreatitis?

Pancreatitis is inflammation of the pancreas. The pancreas is a large gland behind the stomach and close to the duodenum—the first part of the small intestine. The pancreas secretes digestive juices, or enzymes, into the duodenum through a tube called the pancreatic duct. Pancreatic enzymes join with bile—a liquid produced in the liver and stored in the gallbladder—to digest food. The pancreas also releases the hormones insulin and glucagon into the bloodstream. These hormones help the body regulate the glucose it takes from food for energy.

Normally, digestive enzymes secreted by the pancreas do not become active until they reach the small intestine. But when the pancreas is inflamed, the enzymes inside it attack and damage the tissues that produce them.

About This Chapter: This chapter begins with excerpts from "Pancreatitis," National Digestive Diseases Information Clearinghouse (NDDIC), a service of the National Institute of Diabetes and Digestive and Kidney Diseases (NIDDK), July 2008. This chapter also includes excerpts from "Role of Alcohol Metabolism in Chronic Pancreatitis," by Alain Vonlaufen, M.D., and Jeremy S. Wilson, M.D., Romano C. Pirola, M.D., and Minoti V. Apte, Ph.D., *Alcohol Research and Health*, Vol. 30, No. 1, National Institute on Alcohol Abuse and Alcoholism (NIAAA), 2007. The full text of this report, including references, can be found online at http://pubs.niaaa.nih.gov/publications/arh301/48-54.htm.

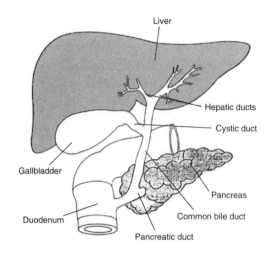

Figure 14.1. The gallbladder and the ducts that carry bile and other digestive enzymes from the liver, gallbladder, and pancreas to the small intestine are called the biliary system.

Pancreatitis can be acute or chronic. Either form is serious and can lead to complications. In severe cases, bleeding, infection, and permanent tissue damage may occur.

The gallbladder and the ducts that carry bile and other digestive enzymes from the liver, gallbladder, and pancreas to the small intestine are called the biliary system.

Both forms of pancreatitis occur more often in men than women.

What is acute pancreatitis?

Acute pancreatitis is inflammation of the pancreas that occurs suddenly and usually resolves in a few days with treatment. Acute pancreatitis can be a life-threatening illness with severe complications. Each year, about 210,000 people in the United States are admitted to the hospital with acute pancreatitis. The most common cause of acute pancreatitis is the presence of gallstones—small, pebble-like substances made of hardened bile—that cause inflammation in the pancreas as they pass through the common bile duct. Chronic, heavy alcohol use is also a common cause. Acute pancreatitis can occur within hours or as long as two days after consuming alcohol. Other causes of acute pancreatitis include abdominal trauma, medications, infections, tumors, and genetic abnormalities of the pancreas.

What is chronic pancreatitis?

Chronic pancreatitis is inflammation of the pancreas that does not heal or improve—it gets worse over time and leads to permanent damage. Chronic pancreatitis, like acute pancreatitis, occurs when digestive enzymes attack the pancreas and nearby tissues, causing episodes of pain. Chronic pancreatitis often develops in people who are between the ages of 30 and 40.

The most common cause of chronic pancreatitis is many years of heavy alcohol use. The chronic form of pancreatitis can be triggered by one acute attack that damages the pancreatic duct. The damaged duct causes the pancreas to become inflamed. Scar tissue develops and the pancreas is slowly destroyed.

Other causes of chronic pancreatitis are listed below.

• Hereditary disorders of the pancreas

• Cystic fibrosis: The most common inherited disorder leading to chronic pancreatitis

♣ It's A Fact!!

It now is generally accepted that alcoholic acute and chronic pancreatitis are the same disease at different stages.

Source: NIAAA, 2007.

• Hypercalcemia: High levels of calcium in the blood

• Hyperlipidemia or hyper-triglyceridemia: High levels of blood fats

• Some medicines

• Certain autoimmune conditions

• Unknown causes

Role Of Alcohol Metabolism In Chronic Pancreatitis

Several theories about how alcohol might lead to pancreatic disease have emerged over the past decades. Whereas early work had predominantly focused on the effects of alcohol on the muscle at the surface of the first part of the small intestine (duodenum), which controls secretions from the liver,

> **♣ It's A Fact!!**
> Alcohol abuse is the major cause of chronic inflammation of the pancreas (chronic pancreatitis). Although it has long been thought that alcoholic pancreatitis is a chronic disease from the outset, evidence is accumulating to indicate that chronic damage in the pancreas may result from repeated attacks of acute tissue inflammation and death (necroinflammation).
>
> Source: National Institute on Alcohol Abuse and Alcoholism (NIAAA), 2007.

pancreas, and gallbladder into the duodenum (the sphincter of Oddi), and on the pancreatic ducts, attention has shifted over the past decade to the influence of alcohol on the clusters of secretory cells (acini) that produce pancreatic juice containing digestive enzymes. Studies with acini or pancreatic acinar cells grown in the laboratory (cultured cells) have established the ability of the pancreas to metabolize alcohol via oxidative and nonoxidative pathways and have provided new insights into the toxic effects of alcohol and the byproducts of its metabolism (metabolites) on the gland. Furthermore, a new era in the understanding of the pathophysiological mechanisms of scar tissue formation in the pancreas (pancreatic fibrosis) has dawned with the recent identification and culture of pancreatic stellate cells (PSCs), the key effector cells in fibrogenesis. Of particular interest is the finding that these cells have the capacity to metabolize alcohol.

Effects Of Alcohol On The Pancreas

Several theories about how alcohol might lead to pancreatic disease have emerged over the past decades. Earlier work had predominantly focused on the effects of alcohol on the muscle at the surface of the first part of the small intestine (duodenum), which controls secretions from the liver, pancreas, and gallbladder into the duodenum (the sphincter of Oddi), and on the pancreatic ducts. Over the past decade, though, attention has shifted to the influence of alcohol on the clusters of secretory cells (acini) that produce pancreatic juice containing digestive enzymes.

Effect Of Alcohol On The Sphincter Of Oddi

Initial research on the effects of alcohol on the pancreas focused on sphincter of Oddi activity. Though, several human studies yielded conflicting results with reports of both decreased and increased sphincter of Oddi activity upon alcohol exposure, ethanol exposure causing spasms has been given more credit by recent evidence in animal studies.

Effects Of Alcohol On Small Ducts: Another theory states that alcohol affects the character of pancreatic fluid to favor the formation of protein plugs and stones. It remains difficult, though, to prove whether ductal stones are a cause or an effect of chronic pancreatitis (CP).

Direct Toxic Effects Of Ethanol On Acinar Cells: In the past decade, the attention of researchers has shifted toward the acinar cells—the most abundant cells in the pancreas. The acinar cell constitutes an "enzyme factory" that produces millions of digestive enzyme molecules every day, and it has been consistently shown in various animal models that one of the first events in acute experimental pancreatitis consists of the premature activation of these enzymes within the acinar cell.

Effect Of Ethanol On Pancreatic Enzymes: Other experimental studies have shown that alcohol consumption leads to an increased amount of digestive and lysosomal enzymes and concurrently increases lysosome and zymogen granule fragility. This is thought to facilitate contact between the lysosomal and digestive enzymes, thereby predisposing the cell to breakdown by its own enzymes, called autodigestion.

Metabolism Of Ethanol By Acinar Cells: Toxic metabolites of ethanol are also known to have adverse effects on several organs in the body. Based on studies in the liver, it is well known that the metabolism of ethanol generates the toxic metabolites acetaldehyde and fatty acid ethyl esters (FAEE), respectively.

Effects Of Toxic Metabolites Of Alcohol: Acetaldehyde and reactive oxygen species (ROS) have also been shown to cause harmful effects on the pancreas. ROS are highly reactive compounds that are potentially harmful to cell membranes, intracellular proteins, and DNA.

☞ Remember!!

- Pancreatitis is inflammation of the pancreas, causing digestive enzymes to become active inside the pancreas and damage pancreatic tissue.

- Pancreatitis has two forms: acute and chronic.

- Common causes of pancreatitis are gallstones and heavy alcohol use.

- Sometimes the cause of pancreatitis cannot be found.

- Symptoms of acute pancreatitis include abdominal pain, nausea, vomiting, fever, and a rapid pulse.

- Treatment for acute pancreatitis includes intravenous (IV) fluids, antibiotics, and pain medications.

- Surgery is sometimes needed to treat complications.

- Acute pancreatitis can become chronic if pancreatic tissue is permanently destroyed and scarring develops.

- Symptoms of chronic pancreatitis include abdominal pain, nausea, vomiting, weight loss, diarrhea, and oily stools.

- Treatment for chronic pancreatitis may involve IV fluids; pain medication; a low-fat, nutritious diet; and enzyme supplements. Surgery may be necessary to remove part of the pancreas.

Source: NIDDK, 2008.

Chapter 15

Alcohol And The Reproductive System

The Effects Of Alcohol On Sexual Function

We know that alcohol affects the body in numerous negative ways. One area that has been widely studied is the effect of alcohol on sexual function. The science is there to explain how and why sexual dysfunction occurs, but that message gets lost when competing for our attention amidst a sea of glitzy alcohol advertising campaigns. Culturally we still hold fast to the notion that alcohol enhances sex. Besides the obvious risk of lowered inhibitions, impaired judgment and resulting bad decision-making while intoxicated, even mild-to-moderate alcohol consumption can produce negative consequences less obvious at the biological level. Alcohol can damage reproductive health in both males and females. Putting aside its relationship with risky sex (risk of sexual assault, sexually transmitted diseases, failure to use contraception, etc.), alcohol can have an enormous effect on our ability to have sex.

In males, inadequate sexual function (hypogonadism) related to alcohol abuse includes testicular atrophy, sterility, impotence, loss of libido, reduction

About This Chapter: This chapter includes information from "The Effects Of Alcohol On Sexual Function," © 2008 National Alliance of Advocates for Buprenorphine Treatment. Reprinted with permission. To view the complete texts, including references, visit www.alcoholanswers.org. Additional information under the heading "Effects Of Alcohol On A Fetus," is from the Substance Abuse and Mental Health Services Administration (SAMHSA), 2007.

in size of the prostate gland, and decreased sperm production. Studies show hypogonadism may be caused both by the direct effects of alcohol on the testis and the effects of alcohol on parts of the brain that regulate gonadal function: the hypothalamus and the pituitary gland. Research suggests that alcohol causes hypogonadism by disrupting the three control points of the hypothalamic-pituitary-gonadal axis (HPG axis, which also refers to the control of ovarian function in the female). Both human and animal studies demonstrate that alcohol consumption is linked to direct toxicity to both the sperm-producing and testosterone-producing cells of the testis. Brain mechanisms that normally compensate to regulate gonadal function are also damaged by alcohol. In layman's terms, alcohol can impair the ability to have and maintain erections as well as the ability to have orgasms.

In females, alcohol use has several negative consequences for reproductive function. Mild-to-moderate alcohol use affects female reproductive function at several stages of life. Studies show that alcohol consumption disrupts female puberty and may also affect growth and bone health. In animal studies with rats, the vaginal opening (a well-characterized marker of puberty in the female rat) was delayed by alcohol administration. Studies show that

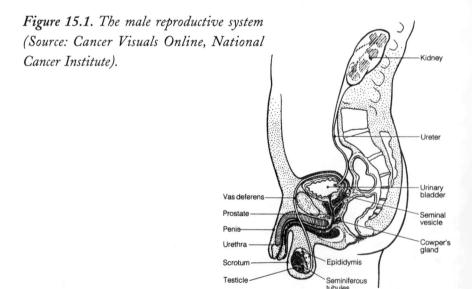

Figure 15.1. The male reproductive system (Source: Cancer Visuals Online, National Cancer Institute).

estrogen levels were decreased among adolescent girls for as long as two weeks after drinking moderately. Because of estrogen's role in bone maturation, it is thought that alcohol use during adolescence may have long-term effects on bone health. Beyond puberty, alcohol can interrupt normal menstrual cycling. Similar to the male, the HPG axis plays a vital role in regulating ovarian function. And like their male counterparts, females experience disrupted hormonal secretions when alcohol is ingested. Alcohol elevates estradiol and temporarily increases testosterone levels, resulting in alterations in estrous cycling. In postmenopausal women the evidence suggests that alcohol exposure affects hormonal levels. Additionally, alcohol inhibits natural lubrication and lowers sensitivity. Common to both males and females, alcohol can impair the ability to have orgasms.

Alcohol plays a big part in our culture and often gets linked to enhanced sexual enjoyment. But the research demonstrates otherwise. The risk of harmful effects on sexual function, as well as growth and bone health, appears especially pronounced during adolescence. However, throughout all life stages there exists the danger that alcohol can impede or impair sexual function.

Figure 15.2. The female reproductive system (Source: Cancer Visuals Online, National Cancer Institute).

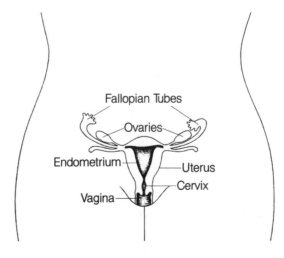

Effects Of Alcohol On A Fetus

What is the scope of the problem?

Alcohol is one of the most dangerous teratogens, which are substances that can damage a developing fetus. Every time a pregnant woman has a drink, her unborn child has one, too. Alcohol, like carbon monoxide from cigarettes, passes easily through the placenta from the mother's bloodstream into her baby's blood—and puts her fetus at risk of having a fetal alcohol spectrum disorder (FASD). The blood alcohol level (BAC) of the fetus becomes equal to or greater than the blood alcohol level of the mother. Because

---

♣ It's A Fact!!
Introduction To The Reproductive System

The major function of the reproductive system is to ensure survival of the species. Other systems in the body, such as the endocrine and urinary systems, work continuously to maintain homeostasis for survival of the individual. An individual may live a long, healthy, and happy life without producing offspring, but if the species is to continue, at least some individuals must produce offspring.

Within the context of producing offspring, the reproductive system has four functions.

• To produce egg and sperm cells

• To transport and sustain these cells

• To nurture the developing offspring

• To produce hormones

These functions are divided between the primary and secondary, or accessory, reproductive organs. The primary reproductive organs, or gonads, consist of the ovaries and testes. These organs are responsible for producing the egg and sperm cells, (gametes), and for producing hormones. These hormones function in the maturation of the reproductive system, the development of sexual characteristics, and have important roles in regulating the normal physiology

the fetus cannot break down alcohol the way an adult can, its BAC remains high for a longer period of time.

What are fetal alcohol spectrum disorders (FASD)?

FASD is an umbrella term describing the range of effects that can occur in an individual whose mother drank alcohol during pregnancy. These effects may include physical, mental, behavioral, and/or learning disabilities with possible lifelong implications. The term FASD is not used as a clinical diagnosis. It refers to conditions such as fetal alcohol syndrome, alcohol-related neurodevelopmental disorder, and alcohol-related birth defects.

of the reproductive system. All other organs, ducts, and glands in the reproductive system are considered secondary, or accessory, reproductive organs. These structures transport and sustain the gametes and nurture the developing offspring.

The Male Reproductive System: The male reproductive system, like that of the female, consists of those organs whose function is to produce a new individual, that is, to accomplish reproduction. This system consists of a pair of testes and a network of excretory ducts (epididymis, ductus deferens—or vas deferens, and ejaculatory ducts), seminal vesicles, the prostate, the bulbourethral glands, and the penis.

The Female Reproductive System: The organs of the female reproductive system produce and sustain the female sex cells (egg cells or ova), transport these cells to a site where they may be fertilized by sperm, provide a favorable environment for the developing fetus, move the fetus to the outside at the end of the development period, and produce the female sex hormones. The female reproductive system includes the ovaries, fallopian tubes, uterus, vagina, accessory glands, and external genital organs.

Source: U.S. National Cancer Institute's Surveillance, Epidemiology and End Results (SEER) Program, 2000. Despite the older date of this document, the anatomical information it provides is still current.

How does alcohol damage a fetus?

Defects caused by prenatal exposure to alcohol have been identified in virtually every part of the body, including the brain, face, eyes, ears, heart, kidneys, and bones. No single mechanism can account for all the problems that alcohol causes. Rather, alcohol sets in motion many processes at different sites in the developing fetus.

♣ **It's A Fact!!**

In the United States, about 130,000 pregnant women each year drink at levels shown to increase the risk of having a child with an FASD. Each year, as many as 40,000 babies are born with an FASD, costing the nation up to $6 billion annually in institutional and medical costs.

Source: Substance Abuse and Mental Health Services Administration (SAMHSA), 2007.

- Alcohol can trigger cell death in a number of ways, causing different parts of the fetus to develop abnormally.

- Alcohol can disrupt the way nerve cells develop, travel to form different parts of the brain, and function.

- By constricting the blood vessels, alcohol interferes with blood flow in the placenta, which hinders the delivery of nutrients and oxygen to the fetus.

- Toxic byproducts of alcohol metabolism may become concentrated in the brain and contribute to the development of an FASD.

♣ **It's A Fact!!**

Although many questions remain unanswered, this much is clear: When a pregnant woman uses alcohol, her baby does too. That's why abstaining from drinking throughout pregnancy and during breastfeeding is the best gift a mother can give her child—it's a gift that lasts a lifetime.

Source: Substance Abuse and Mental Health Services Administration (SAMHSA), 2007.

Drinking at any time during pregnancy can harm the fetus. Drinking alcohol while pregnant can result in cognitive, social, and motor deficiencies and other lifelong problems.

Prenatal exposure to alcohol can cause permanent brain damage. The fetal brain can be harmed at any time, because the brain develops throughout pregnancy. Magnetic resonance imaging (MRI) reveals that some individuals who were prenatally exposed to alcohol have smaller brains. Some parts of the brain may also be damaged or missing, such as the basal ganglia, cerebellum, corpus callosum, and others. Resulting impairments may include, but are not limited to, the following conditions listed below.

- Mental retardation

- Learning disabilities

- Attention deficits

- Hyperactivity

- Problems with impulse control, language, memory, and social skills

Research is under way to learn more about the complex effects of alcohol on a fetus. Increased understanding may lead to improvements in prevention, diagnosis, and treatment of FASD.

♣ **It's A Fact!!**

Prenatal exposure to alcohol can damage a fetus at any time, causing problems that persist throughout the individual's life. There is no known safe level of alcohol use in pregnancy.

Source: Substance Abuse and Mental Health Services Administration (SAMHSA), 2007.

Chapter 16

Facts About Alcohol And Bone Disease

Alcoholism And Recovery

According to the National Institute of Alcohol Abuse and Alcoholism (NIAAA), nearly 14 million Americans—or one in 13 adults—abuse alcohol or are alcoholic. Alcoholism is a disease characterized by a dependency on alcohol. Since alcohol affects almost every organ in the body, chronic heavy drinking is associated with many serious health problems, including pancreatitis, liver disease, heart disease, cancer, and osteoporosis. In fact, the NIAAA estimates that the economic costs of alcohol abuse approach $185 billion per year.

Maintaining sobriety is undoubtedly the most important health goal for an individual recovering from alcoholism. However, attention to other aspects of health, including bone health, can help increase the likelihood of a healthy future, free from the devastating consequences of osteoporosis and fracture.

Facts About Osteoporosis

Osteoporosis is a condition in which bones become less dense and more likely to fracture. Fractures from osteoporosis can result in significant pain

About This Chapter: This chapter includes information from "What People Recovering From Alcoholism Need To Know About Osteoporosis," National Institute of Arthritis and Musculoskeletal and Skin Diseases (NIAMS), August 2005.

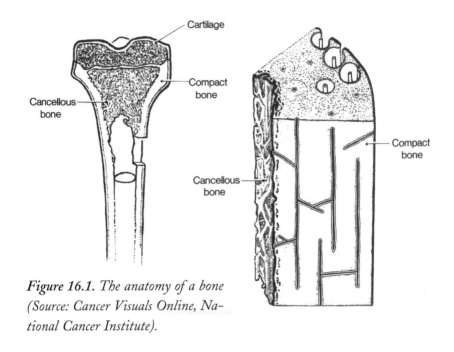

Figure 16.1. The anatomy of a bone (Source: Cancer Visuals Online, National Cancer Institute).

♣ It's A Fact!!

Functions Of The Skeletal System

Humans are vertebrates, animals having a vertebral column or backbone. They rely on a sturdy internal frame that is centered on a prominent spine. The human skeletal system consists of bones, cartilage, ligaments and tendons and accounts for about 20 percent of the body weight.

- **The living bones in our bodies use oxygen and give off waste products in metabolism.** They contain active tissues that consume nutrients, require a blood supply, and change shape or remodel in response to variations in mechanical stress.

- **Bones provide a rigid frame work, known as the skeleton.** The skeleton supports and protects the soft organs of the body. The skeleton supports the body against the pull of gravity. The large bones of the lower limbs support the trunk when standing. The skeleton also protects the soft body parts. The fused bones of the cranium surround the brain to make it less vulnerable to injury. Vertebrae surround and protect the spinal

and disability. It is a major health threat for an estimated 44 million American men and women.

Risk factors for developing osteoporosis include those listed below.

• Being thin or having a small frame

• Having a family history of the disease

• For women, being postmenopausal, having an early menopause, or not having menstrual periods (amenorrhea)

• Using certain medications, such as glucocorticoids

• Not getting enough calcium

• Not getting enough physical activity

• Smoking

• Drinking too much alcohol

cord and bones of the rib cage help protect the heart and lungs of the thorax.

• **Bones work together with muscles.** They act as simple mechanical lever systems to produce body movement.

• **Bones contain more calcium than any other organ.** The intercellular matrix of bone contains large amounts of calcium salts, the most important being calcium phosphate. When blood calcium levels decrease below normal, calcium is released from the bones so that there will be an adequate supply for metabolic needs. When blood calcium levels are increased, the excess calcium is stored in the bone matrix. The dynamic process of releasing and storing calcium goes on almost continuously.

Source: U.S. National Cancer Institute's Surveillance, Epidemiology and End Results (SEER) Program, 2000. Despite the older date of this document, the anatomical information it provides is still current.

♣ It's A Fact!!
Effects Of Moderate and Chronic Heavy Drinking On Bone Health

Moderate Drinking

The effect of moderate alcohol use (federal guidelines consider moderate drinking to be no more than one drink per day for women and no more than two drinks per day for men) on bone health and osteoporosis risk is unclear. A few epidemiological studies in humans have indicated that moderate alcohol consumption may be associated with decreased fracture risk in postmenopausal women. One large study found that women age 65 and over who consumed alcohol on more than five days per week had a significantly reduced risk of vertebral deformity compared with those who consumed alcohol less than once per week. This apparent beneficial effect of moderate drinking on bone health has not been found in animal studies, which can control for the amount of alcohol consumed as well as for other lifestyle factors.

Chronic Heavy Drinking

Effects Of Alcohol On Growing Bone: Almost all epidemiological studies of alcohol use and human bone health indicate that chronic heavy alcohol consumption, particularly during adolescence and young adulthood, can dramatically affect bone health and may increase the risk of developing osteoporosis later. Although alcohol appears to have an effect on bone-forming cells (that is, osteoblasts), slowing bone turnover, the specific mechanisms by which alcohol affects bone are poorly understood.

Studies in female animals have also demonstrated unequivocally that early chronic alcohol consumption compromises bone health, including decrements in bone length, dry weight (weight of the bone with the water removed), and mineral content. Research has shown that young, actively growing rats chronically consuming alcohol had reduced femur lengths when compared with pair-fed control rats until they were approximately nine months of age. Eventually, the femurs of alcohol-fed animals caught up with the growth in length of animals in the control group.

This ability of the femur to make up for lost time, however, did not extend to all measures of bone health. Relative to control animals, alcohol-fed animals' bone density was significantly reduced and remained so throughout the animals' lives.

Effects of Alcohol on Adult Bone: Although alcohol's damaging effects on bone are most striking in young people, research has shown that women between the ages of 67 and 90 who consumed an average of more than three ounces of alcohol per day (the equivalent of six drinks) had greater bone loss than women who had minimal alcohol intake. In addition to such research in human adults, studies of animals that began consuming alcohol as elderly animals also revealed deficiencies in bone volume and density.

Summary

Human and animal studies clearly demonstrate that chronic, heavy alcohol consumption compromises bone health and increases the risk of osteoporosis. In particular, heavy alcohol use decreases bone density and weakens bones' mechanical properties. These effects are particularly striking in young people (and animals), but chronic alcohol use in adulthood can also harm bone health. Further, animal studies suggest that bones do not overcome the damaging effects of early chronic alcohol exposure, even when alcohol use is discontinued.

The effect of moderate alcohol consumption on bone health is less clear. Some research in humans has indicated that moderate drinking may boost bone mass, whereas animal studies have contradicted that idea.

Source: "Alcohol And Other Factors Affecting Osteoporosis Risk In Women," NIAAA, June 2003.

Osteoporosis is a silent disease that can often be prevented. However, if undetected, it can progress for many years without symptoms until a fracture occurs. It has been called "a pediatric disease with geriatric consequences," because building healthy bones in one's youth is important to help prevent osteoporosis and fractures later in life.

♣ **It's A Fact!!**

By about age 35, people reach their peak bone mass. Women lose bone mass slowly after that point until a few years after menopause, when bone mass is lost very rapidly. For middle-aged and older women, healthy bones depend on the development, during younger years, of a strong bone structure and an adequate peak bone mass. There is tenuous evidence that moderate alcohol consumption may protect bone, but human and animal studies clearly indicate that chronic heavy drinking, particularly during adolescence and the young adult years, can dramatically compromise bone quality and may increase osteoporosis risk. Further, research indicates that the effects of heavy alcohol use on bone cannot be reversed, even if alcohol consumption is terminated.

Source: "Alcohol And Other Factors Affecting Osteoporosis Risk In Women," NIAAA, June 2003.

The Alcohol-Osteoporosis Link

Alcohol negatively impacts bone health for several reasons. To begin with, excessive alcohol interferes with the balance of calcium, an essential nutrient for healthy bones. It also increases parathyroid hormone (PTH) levels, which in turn reduce the body's calcium reserves. Calcium balance is further disrupted by alcohol's ability to interfere with the production of vitamin D, a vitamin essential for calcium absorption.

In addition, chronic heavy drinking can cause hormone deficiencies in men and women. Men with alcoholism tend to produce less testosterone, a hormone linked to the production of osteoblasts (the cells that stimulate bone formation). In women, chronic alcohol exposure often produces irregular menstrual cycles, a factor that reduces estrogen levels, increasing osteoporosis risk. Also, cortisol levels tend to be elevated in people with alcoholism. Cortisol is known to decrease bone formation and increase bone breakdown.

Due to the effects of alcohol on balance and gait, people with alcoholism tend to fall more frequently than those without the disorder. Heavy alcohol consumption has been linked to an increase in the risk of fracture, including the most serious kind: hip fracture. Vertebral fractures are also more common in those who abuse alcohol.

Osteoporosis Management Strategies

The most effective strategy for alcohol-induced bone loss is abstinence. People with alcoholism who abstain from drinking tend to have a rapid recovery of osteoblastic (bone building) activity. Some studies have even found that lost bone can be partially restored when alcohol abuse ends.

Nutrition: Due to the negative nutritional effects of chronic alcohol use, people recovering from alcoholism should make healthy nutritional habits a top priority. As far as bone health is concerned, a well-balanced diet rich in calcium and vitamin D is critical. Good sources of calcium include low-fat dairy products; dark green, leafy vegetables; and calcium-fortified foods and beverages. Also, supplements can help ensure that the calcium requirement is met each day. The Institute of Medicine recommends a daily calcium intake of 1,000 mg (milligrams) for men and women, increasing to 1,200 mg for those over age 50.

Vitamin D plays an important role in calcium absorption and bone health. It is synthesized in the skin through exposure to sunlight. Food sources of vitamin D include egg yolks, saltwater fish, and liver. Some individuals may require vitamin D supplements in order to achieve the recommended intake of 400 to 800 IU (International Units) each day.

Exercise: Like muscle, bone is living tissue that responds to exercise by becoming stronger. The best exercise for bones is weight-bearing exercise that forces you to work against gravity. Some examples include walking, climbing stairs, lifting weights, and dancing. Regular exercises such as walking may help prevent bone loss and provide many other health benefits.

Healthy Lifestyle: Smoking is bad for bones as well as the heart and lungs. In addition, smokers may absorb less calcium from their diets. Studies suggest that in people recovering from alcoholism, smoking cessation may actually enhance abstinence from drinking. Since many suspect that smokers who abuse alcohol tend to be more dependent on nicotine than those who don't, a formal smoking cessation program may be a worthwhile investment for individuals in recovery.

Bone Density Test: Specialized tests known as bone mineral density (BMD) tests measure bone density in various sites of the body. These tests can detect osteoporosis before a fracture occurs and predict one's chances of fracturing in the future. Individuals in recovery are encouraged to talk to their health care providers about whether they might be candidates for a bone density test.

Medication: There is no cure for osteoporosis. However, there are medications available to prevent and treat the disease in postmenopausal women and in men.

Chapter 17

Facts About Alcohol And Cancer

Alcohol And Cancer

Cancer kills an estimated 526,000 Americans yearly—second only to heart disease. Cancers of the lung, large bowel, and breast are the most common in the United States. Considerable evidence suggests a connection between heavy alcohol consumption and increased risk for cancer, with an estimated two to four percent of all cancer cases thought to be caused either directly or indirectly by alcohol.

What Is Cancer?

Cancer is a group of diseases characterized by cells that grow out of control. In many cases, they form masses of cells, or tumors, that infiltrate, crowd out, and destroy normal tissue. Although the body strictly regulates normal cells to grow within the confines of tissues, cancer cells reproduce independently, uninhibited by tissue boundaries.

Cancer develops in three stages: initiation, promotion, and progression. Cancer-causing agents, known as carcinogens, can contribute to the first

About This Chapter: This chapter includes information from "Alcohol Alert: Alcohol and Cancer," National Institute on Alcohol Abuse and Alcoholism (NIAAA), October 2000. The complete text of this document, including references, can be found online at http://pubs.niaaa.nih.gov/publications/aa21.htm. The information in this chapter was reviewed for currency by David A. Cooke, M.D., in December 2008.

two stages. Cancer initiation occurs when a cell's DNA (the substance that genes are made of) is irreversibly changed so that, once triggered to divide, the cell will reproduce indefinitely. The change involves mutations to the cell's genes that can occur spontaneously or can be induced by a carcinogen.

In some cancers, it has been shown that the mutations occur in oncogenes, genes that normally promote cell division, or in suppressor genes, genes that normally suppress cell division. Thus, it is believed that cancer-causing mutations result in overpromotion or undersuppression of cell reproduction.

During cancer promotion, the initiated cell is stimulated to divide. The stimulus can be natural, as when tissue damage requires proliferation of new cells, or it can be caused by a carcinogen. During cancer progression, tumors produced by the replicating mass of cells, metastasize (or spread) from the initial or primary tumor to other parts of the body, forming secondary cancers.

> ♣ **It's A Fact!!**
> A strong association exists between alcohol use and cancers of the esophagus, pharynx, and mouth, whereas a more controversial association links alcohol with liver, breast, and colorectal cancers. Together, these cancers kill more than 125,000 people annually in the United States.

Epidemiologic Research

The strongest link between alcohol and cancer involves cancers of the upper digestive tract, including the esophagus, the mouth, the pharynx, and the larynx. Less consistent data link alcohol consumption and cancers of the liver, breast, and colon.

Upper Digestive Tract

Chronic heavy drinkers have a higher incidence of esophageal cancer than does the general population. The risk appears to increase as alcohol consumption increases. An estimated 75 percent of esophageal cancers in the United States are attributable to chronic, excessive alcohol consumption.

Nearly 50 percent of cancers of the mouth, pharynx, and larynx are associated with heavy drinking. People who drink large quantities of alcohol over time have an increased risk of these cancers as compared with abstainers (people who don't drink). If they drink and smoke, the increase in risk is even more dramatic.

Liver

Prolonged, heavy drinking has been associated in many cases with primary liver cancer. However, it is liver cirrhosis, whether caused by alcohol or another factor that is thought to induce the cancer. In areas of Africa and Asia, liver cancer afflicts 50 or more people per 100,000 per year, usually associated with cirrhosis caused by hepatitis viruses. In the United States, liver cancer is relatively uncommon, afflicting approximately two people per 100,000, but excessive alcohol consumption is linked to as many as 36 percent of these cases by some investigators.

The association between alcohol use and liver cancer is difficult to interpret, because liver cirrhosis and hepatitis B and C virus infections often confound the data. Studies of the interactions between alcohol, hepatitis viruses, and cirrhosis will help clarify these associations with liver cancer.

Breast

Chronic alcohol consumption has been associated with a small (averaging 10 percent) increase in a woman's risk of breast cancer. According to

✤ It's A Fact!!
Alcohol's Link To Cancer

Two types of research link alcohol and cancer. Epidemiologic research has shown a dose-dependent association between alcohol consumption and certain types of cancer. For example, as alcohol consumption increases, so does risk of developing certain cancers. More tenuous results have come from research into the mechanism by which alcohol could contribute to cancer development.

these studies, the risk appears to increase as the quantity and duration of alcohol consumption increases. Other studies, however, have found no evidence of such a link.

The inconsistency and weakness of epidemiologic findings suggest that a third confounding factor, such as nutrition, may be responsible for the link between alcohol and breast cancer. However, studies that adjusted for dietary factors, such as fat intake, found that the association between alcohol and breast cancer remained.

♣ **It's A Fact!!**

A few studies have linked chronic heavy drinking with cancers of the stomach, pancreas, and lungs. The association is consistently weak, however, and the majority of studies have found no association.

Recent studies suggest that alcohol may play an indirect role in the development of breast cancer. These studies indicate that alcohol increases estrogen levels in premenopausal women, which, in turn, may promote breast cancer.

Colon

Epidemiologic studies have found a small but consistent dose-dependent association between alcohol consumption and colorectal cancer even when controlling for fiber and other dietary factors. Despite the large number of studies, however, causality cannot be determined from the available data.

Mechanisms Of Alcohol-Related Cancers

The epidemiologic data provide little insight into whether (or how) alcohol increases the risk for various cancers. For some cancers, such as mouth and esophageal, alcohol is thought to play a direct causal role. For others, such as liver and breast cancers, alcohol is thought to play an indirect role by enhancing mechanisms that may cause cancer. Studies looking at these direct and indirect mechanisms may shed light on alcohol's role in developing cancers.

Oncogenes

Preliminary studies show that alcohol may affect cancer development at the genetic level by affecting oncogenes at the initiation and promotion stages of cancer. It has been suggested that acetaldehyde, a product of alcohol metabolism, impairs a cell's natural ability to repair its DNA, resulting in a greater likelihood that mutations causing cancer initiation will occur. It has recently been suggested that alcohol exposure may result in overexpression of certain oncogenes in human cells and, thereby, trigger cancer promotion.

Alcohol As A Cocarcinogen

Although there is no evidence that alcohol itself is a carcinogen, alcohol may act as a cocarcinogen by enhancing the carcinogenic effects of other chemicals. For example, studies indicate that alcohol enhances tobacco's ability to stimulate tumor formation in rats. In humans, the risk for mouth, tracheal, and esophageal cancer is 35 times greater for people who both smoke and drink than for people who neither smoke nor drink, implying a cocarcinogenic interaction between alcohol and tobacco-related carcinogens.

Alcohol's cocarcinogenic effect may be explained by its interaction with certain enzymes. Some enzymes that normally help to detoxify substances that enter the body can also increase the toxicity of some carcinogens. One of these enzymes is called cytochrome P-450. Dietary alcohol is able to induce cytochrome P-450 in the liver, lungs, esophagus, and intestines, where alcohol-associated cancers occur. Subsequently, carcinogens such as those from tobacco and diet can become more potent as they, too, pass through the esophagus, lungs, intestines, and liver and encounter the activated enzyme.

Nutrition

Chronic alcohol abuse may result in abnormalities in the way the body processes nutrients and may subsequently promote certain types of cancer. Reduced levels of iron, zinc, vitamin E, and some of the B vitamins, common in heavy drinkers, have been experimentally associated with some cancers. Also, levels of vitamin A, hypothesized to have anticancer properties, are severely depressed in the liver and esophagus of rats during chronic alcohol consumption.

A recent study indicates that as few as two drinks per day negates any beneficial effects of a correct diet on decreasing risk of colon cancer. Although the study suggests that a diet high in folic acid, a B vitamin found in fresh fruits and vegetables, decreases the risk for colon cancer, it also warns that alcohol consumption may counter this protective action and increase the risk for colon cancer by reducing folic acid levels.

Mechanisms Of Liver Cancer

The possible role of alcohol in the development of liver cancer is incompletely understood. In Asia and Africa, hepatitis B virus infection is thought to cause most liver cancer, though the association is less frequent in the United States. Eighty percent of patients with liver cancer also have cirrhosis, and between 27 and 80 percent test positive for hepatitis B or C infection.

The chronic heavy drinking that causes liver cirrhosis might exacerbate cirrhosis caused independently by the hepatitis B or C viruses. Some studies indicate that alcohol consumption hastens the development of liver cancer in patients with hepatitis C infection, whereas others indicate that alcohol has no compounding effect in such patients.

Suppression Of Immune Response

Alcoholism has been associated with suppression of the human immune system. Immune suppression makes chronic alcohol abusers more susceptible to various infectious diseases and, theoretically, to cancer.

Summary

Although epidemiologic studies have found a clear association between alcohol consumption and development of certain types of cancer, study findings are often inconsistent and may vary by country and by type of cancer. The key to understanding the association lies in research designed to decipher how alcohol may promote cancer. Such studies examine alcohol's metabolic effects at the cellular and genetic levels. Research examining the ways in which alcohol may induce cancers has found some potential mechanisms—the most promising of which implicates oncogenes.

Part Three

Alcohol's Effects On Mental Health And Behavior

Chapter 18

How Alcohol Impacts Memory

Introduction

Alcohol primarily interferes with the ability to form new long-term memories, leaving intact previously established long-term memories and the ability to keep new information active in memory for brief periods. As the amount of alcohol consumed increases, so does the magnitude of the memory impairments.

Large amounts of alcohol, particularly if consumed rapidly, can produce partial (fragmentary) or complete (en bloc) blackouts, which are periods of memory loss for events that transpired while a person was drinking. Blackouts are much more common among social drinkers—including college drinkers—than was previously assumed, and have been found to encompass events ranging from conversations to intercourse.

Mechanisms underlying alcohol-induced memory impairments include disruption of activity in the hippocampus, a brain region that plays a central role in the formation of new autobiographical memories.

About This Chapter: This chapter includes excerpts from "What Happened? Alcohol, Memory Blackouts, And The Brain," by Aaron M. White, Ph.D., *Alcohol Research and Health*, Vol. 27, No. 2, National Institute on Alcohol Abuse and Alcoholism (NIAAA), 2003. The complete text, including references, can be found online at http://pubs.niaaa.nih.gov/publications/arh27-2/186-196.htm.

✦ It's A Fact!!

How does memory work?

To evaluate the effects of alcohol, or any other drug, on memory, one must first identify a model of memory formation and storage to use as a reference. One classic, often-cited model posits that memory formation and storage take place in several stages, proceeding from sensory memory (which lasts up to a few seconds) to short-term memory (which lasts from seconds to minutes depending upon whether the information is rehearsed) to long-term storage. This model often is referred to as the modal model of memory, as it captures key elements of several other major models. Indeed, elements of this model still can be seen in virtually all models of memory formation.

In the modal model of memory, when one attends to sensory information, it is transferred from a sensory memory store to short-term memory. The likelihood that information will be transferred from short-term to long-term storage, or be encoded into long-term memory, was once thought to depend primarily on how long the person keeps the information active in short-term memory via rehearsal. Although rehearsal clearly influences the transfer of information into long-term storage, it is important to note that other factors, such as the depth of processing (that is, the level of true understanding and manipulation of the information), attention, motivation, and arousal also play important roles.

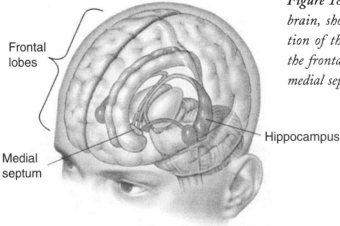

Frontal lobes

Medial septum

Hippocampus

Figure 18.1. The human brain, showing the location of the hippocampus, the frontal lobes, and the medial septum.

Effects Of Alcohol On Memory

Several conclusions can be drawn from research on alcohol-induced memory impairments. One conclusion is that the impact of alcohol on the formation of new long-term "explicit" memories—that is, memories of facts (for example, names and phone numbers) and events—is far greater than the drug's impact on the ability to recall previously established memories or to hold new information in short-term memory.

Intoxicated subjects are typically able to repeat new information immediately after its presentation and often can keep it active in short-term storage for up to a few minutes if they are not distracted, though this is not always the case. Similarly, subjects normally are capable of retrieving information placed in long-term storage prior to acute intoxication. In contrast, alcohol impairs the ability to store information across delays longer than a few seconds if subjects are distracted between the time they are given the new information and the time they are tested.

Intoxicated subjects are typically able to recall information immediately after it is presented and even keep it active in short-term memory for one minute or more if they are not distracted. Subjects also are normally able to recall long-term memories formed before they became intoxicated; however, beginning with just one or two drinks, subjects begin to show impairments in the ability to transfer information into long-term storage. Under some circumstances, alcohol can impact this process so severely that, once sober again, subjects are unable to recall critical elements of events, or even entire events, that occurred while they were intoxicated. These impairments are known as blackouts.

Alcohol-Induced Blackouts

Blackouts represent episodes of amnesia, during which subjects are capable of participating even in salient, emotionally charged events—as well as more mundane events—that they later cannot remember. Like milder alcohol-induced memory impairments, these periods of amnesia are primarily "anterograde," meaning that alcohol impairs the ability to form new memories while the person is intoxicated, but does not typically erase memories formed before intoxication.

Researchers have posited the existence of two qualitatively different types of blackouts: en bloc and fragmentary blackouts. People experiencing en bloc blackouts are unable to recall any details whatsoever from events that occurred while they were intoxicated, despite all efforts by the drinkers or others to cue recall. It is as if the process of transferring information from short-term to long-term storage has been completely blocked. En bloc memory impairments tend to have a distinct onset. It is usually less clear when these blackouts end because people typically fall asleep before they are over. Interestingly, people appear able to keep information active in short-term memory for at least a few seconds. As a result, they can often carry on conversations, drive automobiles, and engage in other complicated behaviors. Information pertaining to these events is simply not transferred into long-term storage.

Unlike en bloc blackouts, fragmentary blackouts involve partial blocking of memory formation for events that occurred while the person was intoxicated. In one study, researchers reported that subjects experiencing fragmentary blackouts often become aware that they are missing pieces of events only after being reminded that the events occurred. Interestingly, these reminders trigger at least some recall of the initially missing information. Research suggests that fragmentary blackouts are far more common than those of the en bloc variety.

Blood Alcohol Concentrations And Blackouts

Drinking large quantities of alcohol often precedes blackouts, but several other factors also appear to play important roles in causing such episodes of memory loss. Among the factors that preceded blackouts were gulping drinks and drinking on an empty stomach, each of which leads to a rapid rise in BAC.

Blackouts Among Social Drinkers

Most of the research conducted on blackouts during the past 50 years has involved surveys, interviews, and direct observation of middle-aged, primarily male alcoholics, many of whom were hospitalized. Researchers have largely ignored the occurrence of blackouts among young social drinkers, so the idea that blackouts are an unlikely consequence of heavy drinking in nonalcoholics has remained deeply entrenched in both the scientific and popular cultures. Yet there is clear evidence that blackouts do occur among social drinkers.

As might be expected given the excessive drinking habits of many college students, this population commonly experiences blackouts. One study surveyed 772 undergraduates regarding their experiences with blackouts (White, AM, et al. Prevalence and correlates of alcohol–induced blackouts among college students: Results of an e-mail survey. *Journal of American College Health* 51:117–131, 2002). Respondents who answered yes to the question "Have you ever awoken after a night of drinking not able to remember things that you did or places that you went?" were considered to have experienced blackouts. Fifty-one percent of the students who had ever consumed alcohol reported blacking out at some point in their lives, and 40 percent reported experiencing a blackout in the year before the survey. Of those who had consumed alcohol during the two weeks before the survey, 9.4 percent reported blacking out during this period. Students in the study reported that they later learned that they had participated in a wide range of events they did not remember, including such significant activities as vandalism, unprotected intercourse, driving an automobile, and spending money.

During the two weeks preceding the survey, an equal percentage of males and females experienced blackouts, despite the fact that males drank significantly more often and more heavily than females. This outcome suggests that at any given level of alcohol consumption, females—a group infrequently studied in the literature on blackouts—are at greater risk than males for experiencing blackouts. The greater tendency of females to black out likely arises, in part, from well-known gender differences in physiological factors that affect alcohol distribution and metabolism, such as body weight, proportion of body fat, and levels of key enzymes. There also is some evidence that females are more susceptible than males to milder forms of alcohol-induced memory impairments, even when given comparable doses of alcohol.

In a subsequent study, researchers interviewed 50 undergraduate students, all of whom had experienced at least one blackout, to gather more information about the factors related to blackouts (White, AM, et. al. Experiential aspects of alcohol–induced blackouts among college students. *American Journal of Drug and Alcohol Abuse*, 2004). As in the previous study, students reported engaging in a range of risky behaviors during blackouts, including sexual activity with both acquaintances and strangers, vandalism, getting into arguments and fights, and others. During the night of their most recent blackout, most students drank either liquor alone or in combination with beer.

Fragmentary blackouts occurred far more often than en bloc blackouts, with four out of five students indicating that they eventually recalled bits and pieces of the events. Roughly half of all students (52 percent) indicated that their first full memory after the onset of the blackout was of waking up in the morning, often in an unfamiliar location. Many students, more females (59 percent) than males (25 percent), were frightened by their last blackout and changed their drinking habits as a result.

Use Of Other Drugs During Blackouts

Alcohol interacts with several other drugs, many of which are capable of producing amnesia on their own. For instance, diazepam (Valium®) and flunitrazepam (Rohypnol) are benzodiazepine sedatives that can produce severe memory impairments at high doses. Alcohol enhances the effects of benzodiazepines. Thus, combining these compounds with alcohol could dramatically increase the likelihood of experiencing memory impairments. Similarly, the combination of alcohol and THC, the primary psychoactive compound in marijuana, produces greater memory impairments than when either drug is given alone.

How Does Alcohol Impair Memory?

During the first half of the 20th century, two theoretical hurdles hampered progress toward an understanding of the mechanisms underlying the effects of alcohol on memory. More recent research has cleared away these hurdles, allowing for tremendous gains in the area during the past 50 years.

The first hurdle concerned scientists' understanding of the functional neuroanatomy of memory. The second barrier to understanding the mechanisms underlying alcohol's effects on memory was an incomplete understanding of how alcohol affects brain function at a cellular level. Until recently, alcohol was assumed to affect the brain in a general way, simply shutting down the activity of all cells with which it came in contact. This view persisted into the late 1980s, at which time the consensus began to shift as evidence mounted that alcohol has selective effects on the brain's nerve-cell communication (neurotransmitter) systems, altering activity in some types of receptors but not others.

♣ It's A Fact!!

Alcohol disrupts activity in the hippocampus via several routes— directly, through effects on hippocampal circuitry, and indirectly, by interfering with interactions between the hippocampus and other brain regions. The impact of alcohol on the frontal lobes remains poorly understood, but probably plays an important role in alcohol-induced memory impairments.

The Role Of Different Brain Regions

More than 30 years ago, researchers speculated that alcohol might impair memory formation by disrupting activity in the hippocampus. This speculation was based on the observation that acute alcohol exposure (in humans) produces a syndrome of memory impairments similar in many ways to the impairments produced by hippocampal damage. Specifically, both acute alcohol exposure and hippocampal damage impair the ability to form new long-term, explicit memories but do not affect short-term memory storage or, in general, the recall of information from long-term storage.

The hippocampus is not the only structure involved in memory formation. Considerable evidence suggests that chronic alcohol use damages the frontal lobes and leads to impaired performance of tasks that rely on frontal lobe functioning. "Shrinkage" in brain volume, changes in gene expression, and disruptions in how performing certain tasks affects blood flow in the brain all have been observed in the frontal lobes of alcohol-dependent subjects.

Although much is known about the effects of chronic (that is, repeated) use of alcohol on frontal lobe function, little is known about the effects of one-time (acute) use of alcohol on activity in the frontal lobes, or the relationship of such effects to alcohol-induced memory impairments. Compelling evidence indicates that acute alcohol use impairs the performance of a variety of frontal lobe-mediated tasks, like those that require planning, decision-making, and impulse control, but the underlying mechanisms are not known. Research also suggests that baseline blood flow to the frontal lobes increases during acute intoxication, that metabolism in the frontal lobes decreases, and that alcohol reduces the amount of activity that occurs in the frontal lobes when the frontal lobes are exposed to pulses from a strong magnetic field. Although the exact meaning of these changes remains unclear, the evidence suggests that acute intoxication alters the normal functioning of the frontal lobes. Future research is needed to shed more light on this important question.

☞ Remember!!

Alcohol can have a dramatic impact on memory. Alcohol primarily disrupts the ability to form new long-term memories. At low doses, the impairments produced by alcohol are often subtle. As the amount of alcohol consumed increases, so does the magnitude of the memory impairments. Large quantities of alcohol, particularly if consumed rapidly, can produce a blackout, an interval of time for which the intoxicated person cannot recall key details of events, or even entire events.

Chapter 19

Binge Drinking, Heavy Drinking, And Blackouts

Binge Drinking

Chet has known Dave since they were in elementary school together, but lately their friendship has been strained. Dave's drinking on weekends has turned him into a completely different person. Dave used to get good grades and play sports, but since he started drinking he hasn't been finishing assignments and he has quit the team.

When Chet saw Dave pound five beers in 30 minutes at two different parties, he realized how serious Dave's problem was. He knows what Dave is doing—binge drinking.

What Is Binge Drinking?

Binge drinking used to mean drinking heavily over several days. Now, however, the term refers to the heavy consumption of alcohol over a short

About This Chapter: This chapter begins with "Binge Drinking," August 2006, reprinted with permission from www.kidshealth.org. Copyright © 2006 The Nemours Foundation. This information was provided by KidsHealth, one of the largest resources online for medically reviewed health information written for parents, kids, and teens. For more articles like this one, visit www.KidsHealth.org or www.TeensHealth.org. Additional text under the heading "Heavy Episodic Consumption of Alcohol," is excerpted from a document of the same name produced by the National Institute on Alcohol Abuse and Alcoholism (NIAAA), September 2005.

period of time (just as binge eating means a specific period of uncontrolled overeating).

Today the generally accepted definition of binge drinking in the United States is the consumption of five or more drinks in a row by men—or four or more drinks in a row by women—at least once in the previous two weeks. Heavy binge drinking includes three or more such episodes in two weeks.

Why Do People Binge Drink?

Liquor stores, bars, and alcoholic beverage companies make drinking seem attractive and fun. It's easy for a high school student to get caught up in a social scene with lots of peer pressure. Inevitably, one of the biggest areas of peer pressure is drinking.

Other reasons why people drink include:

- They're curious—they want to know what it's like to drink alcohol.

- They believe that it will make them feel good, not realizing it could just as easily make them sick and hung-over.

> ♣ **It's A Fact!!**
> **Binge Drinking Affects Non-Drinkers Too**
>
> Non-drinkers may be killed or injured by drunk drivers or by the aggressive actions of someone who has been drinking heavily. Non-drinkers may also find it hard to stay connected to friends or significant others who binge drink because of the changes in that person's behavior.
>
> Source: © 2006 The Nemours Foundation.

- They may look at alcohol as a way to reduce stress, even though it can end up creating more stress.

- They want to feel older.

What Are The Risks Of Binge Drinking?

Many people don't think about the negative side of drinking. Although they think about the possibility of getting drunk, they may not give much consideration to being hung-over or throwing up.

You may know from experience that excessive drinking can lead to difficulty concentrating, memory lapses, mood changes, and other problems that affect your day-to-day life. But binge drinking carries more serious and longer-lasting risks as well.

Alcohol Poisoning

Alcohol poisoning is the most life-threatening consequence of binge drinking. When someone drinks too much and gets alcohol poisoning, it affects the body's involuntary reflexes—including breathing and the gag reflex. If the gag reflex isn't working properly, a person can choke to death on his or her vomit.

> **♣ It's A Fact!!**
>
> **Drinkers At Greater Risk Of Injury:** According to a 2006 Australian study, people who drink are four times more likely than non-drinkers to suffer physical injuries such as falls. And binge drinkers are at an even greater risk of injury.
>
> Source: © 2006 The Nemours Foundation.

Other signs someone may have alcohol poisoning include:

- Extreme confusion
- Inability to be awakened
- Vomiting
- Seizures
- Slow or irregular breathing
- Low body temperature
- Bluish or pale skin

If you think someone has alcohol poisoning, call 911 immediately.

Impaired Judgement

Binge drinking impairs judgement, so drinkers are more likely to take risks they might not take when they're sober. They may drive drunk and injure themselves or others. Driving isn't the only motor skill that's impaired, though. Walking is also more difficult while intoxicated. In 2000, roughly one third of pedestrians 16 and older who were killed in traffic accidents were intoxicated.

People who are drunk also take other risks they might not normally take when they're sober. For example, people who have impaired judgement may have unprotected sex, putting them at greater risk of a sexually transmitted disease (STD) or unplanned pregnancy.

Physical Health

Studies show that people who binge drink throughout high school are more likely to be overweight and have high blood pressure by the time they are 24. Just one regular beer contains about 150 calories, which adds up to a lot of calories if someone drinks four or five beers a night.

♣ **It's A Fact!!**
Drinking And Steroids Don't Mix

Steroids and binge drinking each carry their own health risks. But binge drinking while taking steroids is extremely dangerous. Both alcohol and steroids affect the liver, and combining steroids with drinking can cause liver damage.

Source: © 2006 The Nemours Foundation.

Mental Health

Binge drinkers have a harder time in school and they're more likely to drop out. Drinking disrupts sleep patterns, which can make it harder to stay awake and concentrate during the day. This can lead to struggles with studying and poor academic performance.

People who binge drink may find that their friends drift away—which is what happened with Chet and Dave. Drinking can affect personality; people might become angry or moody while drinking, for example.

Alcoholism

Some studies have shown that people who binge drink heavily—those who have three or more episodes of binge drinking in two weeks—have some of the symptoms of alcoholism.

Getting Help

If you think you or a friend have a binge drinking problem, get help as soon as possible. The best approach is to talk to an adult you trust—if you can't approach your parents, talk to your doctor, school counselor, clergy member, aunt, or uncle.

It can be hard for some people to talk to adults about these issues, so an alternative could be a trusted friend or older sibling who is easy to talk to. Drinking too much can be the result of social pressures, and sometimes it helps to know there are others who have gone through the same thing. If you're worried, don't hesitate to ask someone for help. A supportive friend or adult could help you to avoid pressure situations, stop drinking, or find counseling.

Heavy Episodic Consumption Of Alcohol

In a report titled, "Healthy People 2010" (which sets U.S. public health goals through the year 2010), the Federal government has singled out binge drinking (among college-age students) for a specific, targeted reduction by the year 2010. In the report, they note that binge drinking is a national problem—especially among males and young adults. They also observe that the perception that alcohol use is socially acceptable correlates with the fact that more than 80 percent of American youth consume alcohol before their 21st birthday, whereas the lack of social acceptance of other drugs correlates with comparatively lower rates of use. Similarly, widespread societal expectations that young persons will engage in binge drinking may encourage this highly dangerous form of alcohol consumption.

Understanding Alcohol Consumption

The term alcohol consumption encompasses two ideas important in characterizing an individual's drinking behavior: frequency (how often a person drinks) and quantity (how much a person drinks). Frequency of consumption refers to the number of days or, sometimes, occasions that an individual has consumed alcoholic beverages during a specified interval (for example, week, month, and year). Quantity of consumption refers to the amount ingested on a given drinking occasion.

♣ It's A Fact!!
Blackouts And Memory Lapses

Alcohol can produce detectable impairments in memory after only a few drinks and, as the amount of alcohol increases, so does the degree of impairment. Large quantities of alcohol, especially when consumed quickly and on an empty stomach, can produce a blackout, or an interval of time for which the intoxicated person cannot recall key details of events, or even entire events.

Blackouts are much more common among social drinkers than previously assumed and should be viewed as a potential consequence of acute intoxication regardless of age or whether the drinker is clinically dependent on alcohol. Researchers surveyed 772 college undergraduates about their experiences with blackouts and asked, "Have you ever awoken after a night of drinking not able to remember things that you did or places that you went?" Of the students who had ever consumed alcohol, 51 percent reported blacking out at some point in their lives, and 40 percent reported experiencing a blackout in the year before the survey. Of those who reported drinking in the two weeks before the survey, 9.4 percent said they blacked out during that time. The students reported learning later that they had participated in a wide range of potentially dangerous events they could not remember, including vandalism, unprotected sex, and driving.

Equal numbers of men and women reported experiencing blackouts, despite the fact that the men drank significantly more often and more heavily than the women. This outcome suggests that regardless of the amount of alcohol consumption, females—a group infrequently studied in the literature on blackouts—are at greater risk than males for experiencing blackouts. A woman's tendency to black out more easily probably results from differences in how men and women metabolize alcohol. Females also may be more susceptible than males to milder forms of alcohol-induced memory impairments, even when men and women consume comparable amounts of alcohol.

Source: "Alcohol Alert: Alcohol's Damaging Effects On The Brain," National Institute on Alcohol Abuse and Alcoholism (NIAAA), October 2004.

Most typically, consumption is assessed using "standard drinks." In the United States, these are five ounces of wine, 12 ounces of beer, or 1.25 ounces of distilled spirits. Because individuals do not drink the same amount at every drinking occasion, some surveys attempt to assess the frequency with which a person drinks various amounts of alcohol (for example, one to two drinks, three to four drinks, or five to six drinks) over a specified period of time. Although cumbersome, this approach probably provides a fairly accurate assessment of total volume consumed and of variability in drinking pattern.

For many purposes, however, identifying "light" or "moderate" consumption is not the issue, "heavy" consumption is. For that reason, it is common to assess heavy consumption on the basis of the frequency of consuming a number of drinks meeting or exceeding a certain threshold. Heavy drinking occasions are often referred to as "binges." Researchers define binge drinking as five or more drinks in a row for men and four or more drinks for women.

Historically, binge drinking has referred to an extended period of heavy drinking (for example, a "bender" that lasts three days or more) that is seen in some alcoholic patients. Some clinicians believe that using the term binge to refer to a less severe phenomenon blurs this important distinction.

Other researchers have voiced concern because the specific time period over which the five or four drinks are consumed is not specified nor is the body mass of an individual drinker. For example, after five drinks, consumed over a fixed time span, a man of 240 pounds would have a lower blood alcohol level than a man weighing 140 pounds. Nor would a male or female of the same body weight achieve the same blood alcohol level following equal consumption because of gender-related differences in physiology.

Whether terms such as heavy drinking, binge drinking, or drinking to intoxication are used to describe students' behavior, it is clear that consumption of large quantities of alcohol on a single drinking occasion is important in assessing alcohol involvement. Also key in evaluating alcohol consumption are the consequences of that consumption which can include academic, personal, social, legal, and medical problems as well as dependent symptoms such as tolerance, withdrawal, and loss of control.

♣ It's A Fact!
Binge Drinking And Blackouts

Drinkers who experience blackouts typically drink too much and too quickly, which causes their blood alcohol levels to rise very rapidly. Researchers say that college students may be at particular risk for experiencing a blackout, as an alarming number of them engage in binge drinking. Binge drinking, for a typical adult, is defined as consuming five or more drinks in about two hours for men, or four or more drinks for women.

Source: "Alcohol Alert: Alcohol's Damaging Effects On The Brain," National Institute on Alcohol Abuse and Alcoholism (NIAAA), October 2004.

Chapter 20

Anxiety, Depression, And Suicide Associated With Adolescent Drinking

Depression Symptoms In Childhood Linked To Early Alcohol Use

Kids with moderate to severe symptoms of depression in childhood may be more likely to turn to alcohol in adolescence, according to researchers.

Between 2000 and 2004, the researchers surveyed 1,119 ten- to 13-year-olds and their parents about the child's past and present alcohol use (at the start of the study, none of the children had ever used alcohol). The kids also completed interviews to assess symptoms of depression, anxiety disorders, attention deficit hyperactivity disorder, and substance abuse. They also answered questions about their parents' discipline and monitoring of their activities.

About This Chapter: This chapter begins with "Depression Symptoms In Childhood Linked To Early Alcohol Use," November 2006, reprinted with permission from www.kidshealth.org. copyright © 2006 The Nemours Foundation. This information was provided by KidsHealth, one of the largest resources online for medically reviewed health information written for parents, kids, and teens. For more articles like this one, visit www.TeensHealth.org, or www.KidsHealth.org. Additional information under the headings "Stress, Puberty, And Significant Adolescent Transitions" and "Personality Traits, Mental Disorders, And Adolescent Alcohol Use," is excerpted from *The Surgeon General's Call To Action To Prevent And Reduce Underage Drinking*, Office of the Surgeon General, U.S. Department of Health and Human Services, 2007.

A year or more after the start of the study, nearly 10 percent of kids reported using alcohol. The rate of alcohol use differed significantly, depending on the level of depression symptoms at the start of the study. Among kids who had one or no depression symptoms, about four percent had used alcohol. Of those who reported two to nine depression symptoms, 10 percent had used alcohol. And in kids with 10 or more depression symptoms, fourteen percent had used alcohol.

Kids who were exposed to violence, who displayed antisocial behavior, and who were "thrill seekers" also appeared predisposed to alcohol use. However, those whose parents closely monitored their behaviors and activities appeared to be relatively protected from alcohol use in early adolescence.

What This Means To You

The results of this study indicate that kids who experience depression symptoms in childhood may be more likely to begin using alcohol in adolescence. Other research has shown that early alcohol use is linked to alcohol dependence and addiction later in life. At home, the risks of alcohol use and abuse should be discussed with kids well before adolescence, and parents should teach a variety of strategies for refusing alcohol if it's offered. In addition, children who experience symptoms of depression, such as persistent sadness or hopelessness, extreme irritability or restlessness, or changes in eating or sleeping habits, should talk with their doctors.

Source [of information in reprinted document]: Ping Wu, PhD; Hector R. Bird, MD; Xinhua Liu, PhD; Bin Fan, MD; Cordelia Fuller, MA; Sa Shen, PhD; Cristiane S. Duarte, PhD; Glorisa J. Canino, PhD; *Pediatrics*, November 2006.

Stress, Puberty, And Significant Adolescent Transitions

The physical effects of puberty create dramatic changes in the sexual and social experience of maturing adolescents that require significant psychological and social adaptation. Together with hormonally induced mood and behavior changes, these sexual and social maturation stressors may contribute to increased consumption of alcohol during the adolescent period. In graduating from elementary to middle school, from middle school to high

♣ It's A Fact!!
Substance Use And Suicide Risk

Prior research has associated substance use with an increased risk of suicide among youths. The "2000 National Household Survey on Drug Abuse (NHSDA)" found that youths who reported alcohol or illicit drug use during the past year were more likely than those who did not use these substances to be at risk for suicide during this same time period. For instance, youths who reported past year use of any illicit drug other than marijuana (29 percent) were almost three times more likely than youths who did not (10 percent) to be at risk for suicide during this time period.

Source: Excerpted from "Substance Use And The Risk Of Suicide Among Youths," Substance Abuse and Mental Health Services Administration (SAMHA), 2002.

school, and from high school to college (or the workplace), adolescents move in and out of different social contexts and peer groups, which exposes them to new stressors. These transitions lead to increased responsibilities and academic expectations, which are also potential sources of stress. This is important because research shows a link between stress and alcohol consumption. For example, research on non-human primates shows that adolescent monkeys double their alcohol intake under stress and that excessive alcohol consumption is related to changes in stress hormones and serotonin.

Significant contextual transitions and achievement of milestones for adolescents often occur at specific ages, not at specific developmental periods. For example, the moves to middle and high school and the acquisition of a driver's license and job experience are generally age-based. As a result, some adolescents may be developmentally out of step with the majority of their peers or with the demands of their social environment, particularly in the case of early and late maturing adolescents. A mismatch between social pressures and the cognitive and emotional abilities of an adolescent may increase vulnerability to involvement with alcohol. In the case of early

♣ **It's A Fact!!**

• In 2000, approximately 3 million youths were at risk for suicide during the past year.

• Youths who reported past year alcohol or illicit drug use were more likely than youths who did not use these substances to be at risk for suicide.

• Only 36 percent of youths at risk for suicide during the past year received mental health treatment or counseling.

Source: Excerpted from "Substance Use And The Risk Of Suicide Among Youths," Substance Abuse and Mental Health Services Administration (SAMHA), 2002.

maturing adolescent girls, for example, having an older or adult boyfriend raises the risk for underage use of alcohol and other drugs and the adoption of delinquent behaviors. For boys, same gender peers rather than older romantic interests tend to increase the risk for initiation into alcohol and other drug use. During significant transitions, adolescents can benefit from extra support to avoid alcohol use.

Personality Traits, Mental Disorders, And Adolescent Alcohol Use

Research studies on adolescent drinking have examined the impact of particular personality traits on drinking risk. These studies have repeatedly failed to find specific sets of traits that uniquely predict alcohol use in adolescents. Despite the fact that no set of traits has been found that predicts alcohol use, research does show that adolescents who are heavy alcohol users or have alcohol use disorders (AUDs) often exhibit certain personality traits (which also are shared by some adolescents who do not abuse alcohol). High levels of impulsiveness, aggression, conduct problems, novelty seeking, low harm avoidance, and other risky behaviors in childhood and early adolescence may be associated with future heavy alcohol use and AUDs.

Depression and anxiety also are risk factors for alcohol problems because some people use drinking as a coping strategy for dealing with internal distress. And, more generally, adolescents with defined mental disorders have significantly elevated rates of alcohol and other drug use problems. In these cases, early treatment of mental disorders, such as depression or excessive anxiety, is warranted before an adolescent begins to drink as well as after initiation of drinking. Furthermore, it is important to recognize that youth who use alcohol are also more likely to use other substances and vice versa. Because many young people are involved not only with alcohol but also with other substances and may have a mental disorder, interventions should be designed to address this complexity.

Chapter 21

Alcohol, Violence, And Aggression

It's no secret that alcohol and violence are often related. Many people become aggressive when they drink alcohol, and they are more likely to become violent. Fights and riots in bars and other drinking places remain quite common. In addition, victims of violence often drink as a way of dealing with their pain.

It's important to understand the relationships between alcohol use and violence. Misuse of alcohol and violence can become a cycle, and many people become trapped in it.

Extent Of The Alcohol-Violence Association

Alcohol is quite strongly related to violence. Published statistics report that alcohol use was a factor in up to 86 percent of murders, 37 percent of assaults, and 60 percent of sexual crimes. It was a factor in up to 57 percent of men involved in marital violence and 27 percent of women. In addition, alcohol was a factor in 13 percent of child abusers. In another study, researchers found that 42 percent of violent crimes reported to the police involved alcohol.

About This Chapter: This chapter includes information from "Alcohol Alert: Alcohol, Violence, and Aggression," National Institute on Alcohol Abuse and Alcoholism (NIAAA), October 2000. Reviewed, updated, and adapted for easier reading by David A. Cooke, MD, December 2008.

Alcohol-Violence Relationships

While it's clear that alcohol and violence often go together, scientists are not completely sure why. There are several theories about how one leads to another.

Direct Effects Of Alcohol

Alcohol may encourage aggression or violence by disrupting normal brain function. It's believed that alcohol affects parts of the brain that usually restrain impulsive behaviors and keep aggressiveness under control. Alcohol also interferes with understanding what is seen and heard, which can lead a person to misjudge social cues and overreact. At the same time, alcohol can also prevent understanding the consequences of acting violently.

> ♣ **It's A Fact!!**
> Both alcohol use and violence are common in our society, and there are many associations between the two. Understanding the nature of these associations is essential to developing effective strategies to prevent alcohol-related violence as well as other social problems, such as domestic violence, sexual assault, childhood abuse, and neglect.

Experiments have been performed that show how alcohol affects aggressiveness. In these experiments, a subject gives a test to someone in another room. The tester is given controls and told they can give painful electric shocks as punishments when a mistake is made. In fact, the controls don't really give a shock, but the tester believes that they do.

Some of these experiments have been done on people while sober and repeated after they drink alcohol. In many studies, the more alcohol they drank, the more aggressive the subjects became (for example, by administering stronger shocks).

These findings suggest that alcohol may promote aggressive behavior. However, it's probably more complicated that just a simple equation "alcohol = violence." In the experiments, subjects rarely increased their aggression unless they felt threatened or provoked. Moreover, neither intoxicated nor sober participants administered painful stimuli when other means of communication (for example, a signal lamp) were also available.

These results are consistent with the real-world observation that intoxication alone does not cause violence.

Social And Cultural Expectancies

Alcohol consumption may promote aggression because people expect it to. For example, research using real and fake alcoholic beverages shows that people who believe they have consumed alcohol begin to act more aggressively, regardless of which beverage they actually consumed. The expectation that men will become more aggressive after alcohol, combined with the widespread perception of intoxicated women as being more open to sex and less able to defend themselves, could account for the association between drinking and date rape.

In addition, a person who intends to engage in a violent act may drink to bolster his or her courage or in hopes of evading punishment. There is a popular view of intoxication as a "time-out," during which one is not subject to the same rules of conduct as when sober.

Violence Preceding Alcohol Misuse

Childhood Victimization

A history of childhood sexual abuse or neglect is more likely among women with alcohol problems than among women without alcohol problems. However, researchers found no relationship between childhood victimization and subsequent alcohol misuse in men. Even children who only witness family violence may learn to imitate it, setting the stage for alcohol abuse and violence to persist over generations. Finally, alcohol-related brain damage before birth, combined with subsequent parental neglect such as might occur in an alcoholic family, may predispose one to violence, crime, and other behavioral problems by age 18.

Violent Lifestyles

Violence may precede alcohol misuse in offenders as well as victims. For example, violent people may be more likely than nonviolent people encounter social situations that encourage heavy drinking. In summary, violence may lead to alcohol consumption, which in turn may lead to more violence.

Common Causes For Alcohol Misuse And Violence

In many cases, abuse of alcohol and a propensity to violence may stem from a common cause. This cause may be due to a risk-seeking personality, or a social environment that encourages or contributes to deviant behavior.

Another example of a common cause relates to the frequent co-occurrence of antisocial personality disorder (ASPD) and early-onset (that is, type 2) alcoholism. ASPD is a psychiatric disorder characterized by a disregard for the rights of others, often manifested as a violent or criminal lifestyle. Type 2 alcoholism is characterized by high heritability from father to son; early onset of alcoholism (often during adolescence); and antisocial, sometimes violent, behavioral traits. Type 2 alcoholics and persons with ASPD overlap in their tendency to violence and excessive alcohol consumption and may share a genetic basis.

Spurious Associations

Spurious (that is, coincidental) associations between alcohol consumption and violence may arise by chance or coincidence, with no direct or common cause. For example, drinking is a common social activity for many adult Americans, especially those most likely to commit violent acts. Therefore, drinking and violence may occur together by chance. In addition, violent criminals who drink heavily are more likely than less intoxicated offenders to be caught and consequently are over-represented in samples of convicts or arrestees. Spurious associations may sometimes be difficult to distinguish from common-cause associations.

> ♣ **It's A Fact!!**
> Understanding more about alcohol-related violence will also shed light on violence in general and produce information that may be useful to reducing it.

Physiology Of Violence

Although individual behavior is shaped in part by the environment, it is also influenced by biological factors (for example, hormones) and ultimately planned and directed by the brain. Individual differences in brain chemistry may explain the observation that excessive alcohol consumption may consistently promote aggression in some persons, but not in others. The following subsections highlight some areas of intensive study.

Serotonin

Serotonin, a chemical messenger in the brain, is thought to function as a behavioral inhibitor. Thus, decreased serotonin activity is associated with increased impulsivity and aggressiveness as well as with early-onset alcoholism among men.

Experiments in animals can simulate many of the characteristics of alcoholism in humans. Rhesus macaque monkeys sometimes consume alcohol in sufficient quantities to become intoxicated. Monkeys with low serotonin activity consume alcohol faster; these monkeys also demonstrate impaired impulse control, with excessive and inappropriate aggression. This behavior and brain chemistry closely resemble that of type 2 alcoholics. Interestingly, among both monkeys and humans, parental neglect leads to early-onset aggression and excessive alcohol consumption in the offspring, again correlated with decreased serotonin activity.

Although data are inconclusive, the alcohol-violence link may be mediated by chemical messengers in addition to serotonin, such as dopamine and norepinephrine. There is also considerable overlap among nerve cell pathways in the brain that regulate aspects of aggression, sexual behavior, and alcohol consumption. This suggests a biological reason for the frequent co-occurrence of alcohol intoxication and sexual violence.

Testosterone

The steroid hormone testosterone is responsible for the development of male sexual characteristics. High testosterone concentrations in criminals have been associated with violence, suspiciousness, and hostility. In animal experiments, alcohol administration increased aggressive behavior in socially dominant squirrel monkeys, who already exhibited high levels of aggression and testosterone. Alcohol did not, however, increase aggression in lower-ranking monkeys, which exhibited low levels of aggression and testosterone.

These findings may shed some light on the life cycle of violence in humans. In humans, violence mostly occurs among adolescent and young adult males, who tend to have high levels of testosterone. Young men who exhibit antisocial behaviors often "burn out" with age, becoming less aggressive when they reach their forties. By that age, testosterone concentrations are decreasing, while serotonin concentrations are increasing, both factors that tend to restrain violent behavior.

Conclusion

No one model can account for all individuals or types of violence. Alcohol apparently may increase the risk of violent behavior only for certain people and only under some situations.

Although much remains to be learned, research suggests that some violent behavior may be treatable or preventable. One study found decreased levels of marital violence in couples who completed behavioral marital therapy for alcoholism and remained sober during follow-up. Results of another study suggest that a 10 percent increase in the beer tax could reduce murder by 0.3 percent, rape by 1.32 percent, and robbery by 0.9 percent. Although these results are modest, they indicate a direction for future research. In addition, preliminary experiments have identified medications that have the potential to reduce violent behavior. Such medications include certain anticonvulsants (for example, carbamazepine); mood stabilizers (for example, lithium); and antidepressants, especially those that increase serotonin activity (for example, fluoxetine).

> **☞ Remember!!**
>
> Understanding the biology of violence will help us to clearly define the role of the environment in increasing the risk for violence and increase our understanding of who is at risk for violent behavior. This understanding also will help us to develop effective interventions—both social and medical—to help those whose violence has caused trouble for themselves and others.

Chapter 22

Overconfidence And Recklessness Associated With Adolescent Drinking

Underage Drinking

Underage drinkers experience a wide range of alcohol-related health, social, criminal justice, and academic problems. They do not all experience the same level of problems–those who drink more, and drink more often, suffer a greater number of negative consequences. However, negative consequences occur across a wide range of consumption levels and frequencies.

Young drinkers report a range of negative effects from alcohol, all of which can lead to troubled interactions with others, particularly police officers or other responsible adults who try to intervene. These include the following:

- **Overconfidence And Recklessness:** Excessive drinking may cause people to act in ways they would normally consider unwise or inappropriate.

About This Chapter: This chapter includes excerpts from the *Problem-Oriented Guides for Police Problem-Specific Guides Series, No. 27,* "Underage Drinking," by Kelly Dedel Johnson, September 2004. This project was supported by cooperative agreement #2002CKWX0003 by the Office of Community Oriented Policing Services, U.S. Department of Justice.

Risks

♣ **It's A Fact!!**

Alcohol use among youth is strongly correlated with violence, risky sexual behavior, poor academic performance, and other harmful behaviors.

Violence

• Children who start drinking before age 15 are 12 times more likely to be injured while under the influence of alcohol and 10 times more likely to be in a fight after drinking, compared with those who wait until they are 21.

Sexual Activity

• Alcohol use by teens is a strong predictor of both sexual activity and unprotected sex.

• A survey of high school students found that 18% of females and 39% of males say it is acceptable for a boy to force sex if the girl is high or drunk.

School

• Teens who use alcohol have higher rates of academic problems and poor performance than non-drinkers.

• Among eighth-graders, higher truancy rates are associated with greater rates of alcohol use in the past month.

Illicit Drug Use

• More than 67% of young people who start drinking before the age of 15 will try an illicit drug. Children who drink are 7.5 times more likely to use any illicit drug, more than 22 times more likely to use marijuana, and 50 times more likely to use cocaine than children who never drink.

Driving

• When young people drink and get into a car, they tend to make poor decisions that impact their safety.

• Traffic crashes are the number one killer of teens and over one-third of teen traffic deaths are alcohol-related.

Source: "Start Talking Before They Start Drinking: A Family Guide," Substance Abuse and Mental Health Services Admin. (SAMHSA), Center for Substance Abuse Prevention, 2006.

- **Lack Of Awareness:** As people become intoxicated, they may not be fully aware of what is happening, and they may not be able to figure out how to react to situations appropriately.

- **Aggression:** Drinkers may misread cues from other people as being offensive and react violently.

- **Loss Of Control:** Drinkers' motor skills may become impaired, and drinkers may also lose control of their emotions.

These effects often lead young drinkers to come into contact with police, either as offenders or as victims. Youths who drink heavily are more likely to carry handguns than those who do not drink. Alcohol use contributes to property damage, rape, and other violent crime on college campuses, and about half of college crime victims have been drinking before the crime occurs. A significant proportion of young drivers killed in car accidents are intoxicated when the crash occurs.

Further, underage college students who drink heavily are more likely to miss class, fall behind in school, sustain an injury, have unplanned or unprotected sex, drive after drinking, or have contact with campus police. Students also experience "secondhand" effects of others' alcohol misuse, such as having their sleep or study time interrupted; having to take care of an intoxicated friend; being insulted or humiliated by drinkers; receiving unwanted sexual advances; getting in serious arguments; having their personal property damaged; being assaulted, sexually or otherwise; and being raped by an acquaintance. There are also a number of physical and mental health-related consequences of alcohol use, which are detailed elsewhere.

Very few college students experience any college-based disciplinary action as a result of their drinking, despite widespread use and serious consequences for the individuals, their peers, and their communities. The past decade has witnessed increased concern about and creativity in confronting the issue, and both adults and youths support measures to prevent underage drinking. Given the issue's complexity, it is important to understand how the problem takes shape in your community. Analyzing the factors that contribute to your local underage drinking problem will help you to select the most effective responses.

Related Problems

Underage drinking is associated with a number of other problems not directly addressed in this chapter. These related problems require their own analyses and responses:

- Drunken driving

- Speeding in residential areas

- Cruising

- Disorderly conduct in public places

- Assaults in and around bars

- Acquaintance rape

- House parties

- Rave parties

- Vandalism

- Noise complaints in residential areas

♣ **It's A Fact!!**

Alcohol And Judgement

The teenage brain is still developing, and alcohol can impair the parts of the brain.

- **Motor Coordination:** This includes the ability to walk, drive, and process information.

- **Impulse Control:** Drinking lowers inhibitions and increases the chances that a person will do something that they will regret when they are sober.

- **Memory:** Impaired recollection and even blackouts can occur when too much alcohol has been consumed.

- **Judgement And Decision-Making Capacity:** Drinking may lead young people to engage in risky behaviors that can result in illness, injury, and even death.

Source: "Start Talking Before They Start Drinking: A Family Guide," Substance Abuse and Mental Health Services Admin. (SAMHSA), Center for Substance Abuse Prevention, 2006.

Chapter 23

Drinking And Sexual Risk Taking

Does this situation sound familiar to you?

> Denise: "Are you going to Steve's party Friday night? I hear they will have a lot of booze there . . . and best of all, no adults! I think he has the hots for me! He always compliments my outfits I wear to school."

> Kelcey: "Denise, the guy does that to every girl in our school. You are not special to him. Besides, I hear he is dating someone."

> Denise: "So what, he says I have beautiful eyes. Secretly, we've been kissing everyday this week after gym class. If all goes well, according to him, after Friday night's party, we will really be boyfriend and girlfriend."

> Kelcey: "What does that mean? I hope you don't plan on doing it with him! Please don't fall for that trick. I won't be going to that party and you shouldn't either!" said Kelcey.

About This Chapter: This chapter begins with excerpts from "Abstinence—Safe Sex Is No Sex," Office on Women's Health, U.S. Department of Health and Human Services (DHHS), June 18, 2008. "Some Facts about Teens and Sex," is from the DHHS website 4Parents.gov, November 13, 2007. "Some Facts about Underage Drinking and Risky Sexual Behavior" is excerpted from "Steep Risks When Youth Drink," *Prevention Alert*, National Clearinghouse for Alcohol and Drug Information, Substance Abuse and Mental Health Services Administration, January 23, 2003.

You may have played the role of Denise or Kelcey: A cute guy from your school invites you to a party with plenty of alcohol and no adults. Everyone that's anyone will be there. How can you possibly say no? Then, of course, there is the cute guy, Steve—who has been flirting with you all week at school. This is probably your one opportunity to show him how much you like him. You can't let him down and miss this party. He'll never speak to you again!

One problem—your friend, Kelcey. She opposes this party with good reason. No adults, plenty of alcohol, sounds like trouble to her, spelled S-E-X. Too bad you are too "starry eyed" to figure this one out. Kelcey thinks Steve is bad news. She has good reason. He's hit on her a couple of times. His reputation with girls at school is not one to be admired.

The thought of having sex while you are a teenager may seem pretty cool and a really good way to get someone to like you, but it can backfire. The truth is, having sex while you are a teen can make you feel bad about yourself and your partner. While sex may look like something very attractive and worthwhile, you often don't see what can happen after sex when you are a teen.

Just Saying "No" Is Not Always Easy

Abstinence doesn't just happen. Saying "no" to sexual intercourse, mutual masturbation, and oral sex is not enough. You have to think about it ahead of time, make a plan, follow through, and have support from parents, friends, and people you trust. Get clear about why you've made the choice to be

---

✤ It's A Fact!!

- Current teen drinkers are more than twice as likely to have had sexual intercourse within the past three months than teens who don't drink.

- Higher drinking levels increase the likelihood of sexual activity.

- Adolescents who drink are more likely to engage in risky sexual activities, like having sex with someone they don't know or failing to use birth control.

Source: Excerpted from "Dangers of Teen Drinking," Federal Trade Commission (FTC), March 2008.

abstinent, and talk to your partner about what you want and don't want and why. Don't be afraid to take a stand about your decision. If you and your partner can't agree, then maybe you need to find someone whose beliefs are closer to your own.

Keep in mind, you are more than just a body. During your junior and senior high school years, you may be strongly attracted to a cute guy, such as Steve. Your body may send you strong messages that make you want to get closer to him. Be sure to think before you act. Think about your future. Think about what may happen if you have sex. Your body won't tell you how having sex may harm you physically, emotionally, socially, spiritually, and financially.

♣ It's A Fact!!

Adolescents are more likely to engage in high-risk behaviors, such as unprotected sex, when they are under the influence of drugs or alcohol. In 2007, 23% of high school students who had sexual intercourse during the past three months drank alcohol or used drugs before last sexual intercourse.

Source: "Sexual Risk Behaviors," National Center for Chronic Disease Prevention and Health Promotion, October 23, 2008.

Good relationships don't develop overnight. They take time. Think about your goals and your partner's goals—graduating from high school, going to college, and starting a career. Instead of focusing on sex join the band, a sports team, or the school choir; get involved with community or faith-based organizations; look for summer programs and internships; or help others in your community.

Keep in mind, sex is NOT what makes a relationship work. If you are confronted with this line— "If you care about me, you'll have sex with me" —don't believe it. You don't have to have sex with someone to prove you like or love him. Sharing time, thoughts, beliefs, feelings, and mutual respect is what makes a relationship strong. Saying "no" can be the best way to say, "I love you." It is always best to make the choice to wait.

♣ It's A Fact!!
The Emotional Risks Of Early Sexual Activity

People often believe that the only risks from teens having sex are pregnancy or getting a sexually transmitted disease (STD). Not true. Teens who have sex are at risk for emotional problems too.

It has been clear for quite some time that teen sex and emotional problems such as depression are related. What has not been clear is if teen sex causes depression, or depression causes teens to have sex. Recent research suggests that both may be true. Teens, especially girls, who have sexual intercourse may be at greater risk for depression. And depression in teens is now known to lead to risky sexual behaviors.

A 2005 study recommended that teen girls who have sex be screened for depression. This journal article found that teen girls who had sex, took drugs, and/or started drinking were up to three times more likely to be depressed a year later than girls who did not take those risks.

For boys, the researchers found things to be a bit different. Boys who do a number of unhealthy things, like smoking cigarettes every day, smoking marijuana, and drinking alcohol, were more likely to be depressed.

Another study, which also used data from that same large survey of teens, tried to learn whether depression predicts risky sexual behavior. The researchers found that boys and girls who have symptoms of depression are more likely to get involved in very risky sexual behaviors, such as not using a condom, having sex with a number of partners, and using alcohol or other drugs when they had sex.

One thing is also very clear: most teens who have sex wish they had waited. In fact, whether you ask boys or girls, older teens or younger teens, a large majority say they wish they had waited. According to a survey conducted by the National Campaign to Prevent Teen Pregnancy, two out of three (66%) sexually experienced teens wish they had waited longer before first having sexual intercourse. And nearly two out of three (63%) of those teen boys and more than two out of three (69%) of those teen girls wish they had waited. And of those teens 12- to 14-years-old, seven out of ten (71%) wish they had waited. Of those teens 15–19, six out of ten (63%) said they wish they had waited.

Source: U.S. Department of Health and Human Services, May 13, 2008. This document, with links to resources, is available online at http://www.4parents.gov/sexrisky/emotional/emotional.html.

Some Facts About Teens And Sex

You may be surprised to know that most high school students have not had sexual intercourse. That's right, 53% of all high school students have not had sexual intercourse. And it's not much different for boys and girls. That 53% breaks down to 54% of high school girls and 52% of high school boys.

Teens who have sex are at high risk for pregnancy and sexually transmitted diseases (STDs). Nearly one out of every three (31%) teen girls who have had sexual experience have been pregnant while still teens. More then one out of every eight (13%) teen boys who have had sexual experience have gotten a girl pregnant while still teens. And teens and young adults who have sex get one out of every two (50%) new STD infections each year.

The younger a teen starts having sex, the greater the risk of pregnancy. Of girls who first have sex before age 15, almost half of them will get pregnant. Girls who have had three or more sexual partners are more likely to get pregnant, as well. Plus, the more sexual partners a person has over time, the more likely he or she is to get an STD. One out of seven (14%) high school students report having had sex with four or more partners.

Some Facts About Underage Drinking And Risky Sexual Behavior

Underage drinking is linked to an increase in risky sexual behavior. According to a national survey of sexually active young people, 12 percent of teens aged 15 to 17 reported having unprotected sex as a result of having been drinking or using drugs. In addition, 24 percent reported that because of their substance use, they had "done more" sexually than they had planned.

Teenage girls who are heavy drinkers are five times more likely than non-drinkers to engage in sexual intercourse and a third less likely to use condoms, which can result in pregnancy and sexually transmitted diseases.

Chapter 24

Drinking And Date Rape Drugs

What are date rape drugs?

These are drugs that are sometimes used to assist a sexual assault. Sexual assault is any type of sexual activity that a person does not agree to. It can include touching that is not okay; putting something into the vagina; sexual intercourse; rape; and attempted rape. These drugs are powerful and dangerous. They can be slipped into your drink when you are not looking. The drugs often have no color, smell, or taste, so you can't tell if you are being drugged. The drugs can make you become weak and confused—or even pass out—so that you are unable to refuse sex or defend yourself. If you are drugged, you might not remember what happened while you were drugged. Date rape drugs are used on both females and males.

These are the three most common date rape drugs:

- **Rohypnol** (roh-HIP-nol): Rohypnol is the trade name for flunitrazepam (FLOO-neye-TRAZ-uh-pam). Abuse of two similar drugs appears to have replaced Rohypnol abuse in some parts of the United States. These are clonazepam (marketed as Klonopin in the U.S. and Rivotril in Mexico) and alprazolam (marketed as Xanax).

About This Chapter: From "Frequently Asked Questions: Date Rape Drugs," Office on Women's Health, U.S. Department of Health and Human Services, May 1, 2007.

- **GHB**, which is short for gamma hydroxybutyric (GAM-muh heye-DROX-ee-BYOO-tur-ihk) acid

- **Ketamine** (KEET-uh-meen)

These drugs also are known as "club drugs" because they tend to be used at dance clubs, concerts, and "raves." They go by many street names:

Rohypnol: Circles; Lunch Money; Poor Man's Quaalude; Roach; Roofies; Rophies; Whiteys; Forget Pill; Mexican Valium; R-2; Roach-2; Roopies; Ruffies; LA Rochas; Mind Erasers; Rib; Roches; Rope; Trip-and-Fall

GHB: Bedtime Scoop; Energy Drink; Gamma 10; Goop; Liquid E; PM; Somatomax; Cherry Meth; G; Georgia Home Boy; Great Hormones; Liquid Ecstasy; Salt Water; Vita-G; Easy Lay; G-Juice; Gook; Grievous Bodily Harm (GBH); Liquid X; Soap

Ketamine: Black Hole; Green; K-Hole; Purple; Bump; Jet; Kit Kat; Special K; Cat Valium; K; Psychedelic Heroin; Super Acid

What do the drugs look like?

Rohypnol comes as a pill that dissolves in liquids. Some are small, round, and white. Newer pills are oval and green-gray in color. When slipped into a drink, a dye in these new pills makes clear liquids turn bright blue and dark drinks turn cloudy. But this color change might be hard to see in a dark drink, like cola or dark beer, or in a dark room. Also, the pills with no dye are still available. The pills may be ground up into a powder.

GHB has a few forms: a liquid with no odor or color, white powder, and pill. It might give your drink a slightly salty taste. Mixing it with a sweet drink, such as fruit juice, can mask the salty taste.

Ketamine comes as a liquid and a white powder.

What effects do these drugs have on the body?

These drugs are very powerful. They can affect you very quickly and without your knowing. The length of time that the effects last varies. It depends on how much of the drug is taken and if the drug is mixed with other drugs or alcohol. Alcohol makes the drugs even stronger and can cause serious health problems—even death.

Rohypnol: The effects of Rohypnol can be felt within 30 minutes of being drugged and can last for several hours. If you are drugged, you might look and act like someone who is drunk. You might have trouble standing. Your speech might be slurred. Or you might pass out. Rohypnol can cause these problems:

- Muscle relaxation or loss of muscle control
- Difficulty with motor movements
- Drunk feeling
- Problems talking
- Nausea
- Can't remember what happened while drugged
- Loss of consciousness (blackout)
- Confusion
- Problems seeing
- Dizziness
- Sleepiness
- Lower blood pressure
- Stomach problems
- Death

GHB: GHB takes effect in about 15 minutes and can last three or four hours. It is very potent: A very small amount can have a big effect. So it's easy to overdose on GHB. Most GHB is made by people in home or street "labs." So, you don't know what's in it or how it will affect you. GHB can cause these problems:

- Relaxation
- Drowsiness
- Dizziness
- Nausea
- Problems seeing
- Loss of consciousness (blackout)
- Seizures
- Can't remember what happened while drugged
- Problems breathing
- Tremors
- Sweating
- Vomiting
- Slow heart rate
- Dream-like feeling
- Coma
- Death

Ketamine: Ketamine is very fast-acting. You might be aware of what is happening to you, but unable to move. It also causes memory problems. Later, you might not be able to remember what happened while you were drugged. Ketamine can cause these problems:

- Distorted perceptions of sight and sound
- Lost sense of time and identity
- Out of body experiences
- Dream-like feeling
- Feeling out of control
- Impaired motor function
- Problems breathing
- Convulsions
- Vomiting
- Memory problems
- Numbness
- Loss of coordination
- Aggressive or violent behavior
- Depression
- High blood pressure
- Slurred speech

Are these drugs legal in the United States?

Some of these drugs are legal when lawfully used for medical purposes. But that doesn't mean they are safe. These drugs are powerful and can hurt you. They should only be used under a doctor's care and order.

Rohypnol is NOT legal in the United States. It is legal in Europe and Mexico, where it is prescribed for sleep problems and to assist anesthesia before surgery. It is brought into the United States illegally.

Ketamine is legal in the United States for use as an anesthetic for humans and animals. It is mostly used on animals. Veterinary clinics are robbed for their ketamine supplies.

GHB was recently made legal in the United States to treat problems from narcolepsy (a rare sleep disorder). Distribution of GHB for this purpose is tightly restricted.

Is alcohol a date rape drug? What about other drugs?

Any drug that can affect judgment and behavior can put a person at risk for unwanted or risky sexual activity. Alcohol is one such drug. In fact, alcohol is the drug most commonly used to help commit sexual assault. When a person drinks too much alcohol:

- It's harder to think clearly.

- It's harder to set limits and make good choices.

- It's harder to tell when a situation could be dangerous.

- It's harder to say "no" to sexual advances.

- It's harder to fight back if a sexual assault occurs.

- It's possible to blackout and to have memory loss.

♣ **It's A Fact!!**

The term "date rape" is widely used. But most experts prefer the term "drug-facilitated sexual assault." These drugs also are used to help people commit other crimes, like robbery and physical assault. They are used on both men and women. The term "date rape" also can be misleading because the person who commits the crime might not be dating the victim. Rather, it could be an acquaintance or stranger.

The club drug "ecstasy" (MDMA) has been used to commit sexual assault. It can be slipped into someone's drink without the person's knowledge. Also, a person who willingly takes ecstasy is at greater risk of sexual assault. Ecstasy can make a person feel "lovey-dovey" towards others. It also can lower a person's ability to give reasoned consent. Once under the drug's influence, a person is less able to sense danger or to resist a sexual assault.

How can I protect myself from being a victim?

- Don't accept drinks from other people.

- Open containers yourself.

- Keep your drink with you at all times, even when you go to the bathroom.

- Don't share drinks.

- Don't drink from punch bowls or other common, open containers. They may already have drugs in them.

✔ **Quick Tip**

For more information on date rape drugs, please call the Office on Women's Health (http://www.womenshealth.gov) at 800-994-9662 or contact the following organizations:

Drug Enforcement Administration, Department of Justice
Phone: 202-307-1000
Website: http://www.usdoj.gov/dea

Food and Drug Administration
Phone: 800-332-4010 (Hotline) or 888-463-6332 (Consumer Information)
Website: http://www.fda.gov

Men Can Stop Rape
Phone: 202-265-6530
Website: http://www.mencanstoprape.org

National Center for Victims of Crime
Phone: 800-394-2255
Website: http://www.ncvc.org

National Institute on Drug Abuse
Phone: 800-662-4357 (Hotline) or 800-662-9832 (Spanish Language Hotline)
Website: http://www.drugabuse.gov

Office of National Drug Control Policy
Phone: 800-666-3332 (Information Clearinghouse)
Website: http://www.whitehousedrugpolicy.gov

Rape, Abuse, and Incest National Network
Phone: 800-656-4673 (800-656-HOPE)
Website: http://www.rainn.org

- If someone offers to get you a drink from a bar or at a party, go with the person to order your drink. Watch the drink being poured and carry it yourself.

- Don't drink anything that tastes or smells strange. Sometimes, GHB tastes salty.

- Have a nondrinking friend with you to make sure nothing happens.

- If you realize you left your drink unattended, pour it out.

- If you feel drunk and haven't drunk any alcohol—or, if you feel like the effects of drinking alcohol are stronger than usual—get help right away.

Are there ways to tell if I might have been drugged and raped?

It is often hard to tell. Most victims don't remember being drugged or assaulted. The victim might not be aware of the attack until eight or 12 hours after it occurred. These drugs also leave the body very quickly. Once a victim gets help, there might be no proof that drugs were involved in the attack. But there are some signs that you might have been drugged:

- You feel drunk and haven't drunk any alcohol—or, you feel like the effects of drinking alcohol are stronger than usual.

- You wake up feeling very hung over and disoriented or having no memory of a period of time.

- You remember having a drink, but cannot recall anything after that.

- You find that your clothes are torn or not on right.

- You feel like you had sex, but you cannot remember it.

What should I do if I think I've been drugged and raped?

Get medical care right away. Call 911 or have a trusted friend take you to a hospital emergency room. Don't urinate, douche, bathe, brush your teeth, wash your hands, change clothes, or eat or drink before you go. These things may give evidence of the rape. The hospital will use a "rape kit" to collect evidence.

Call the police from the hospital. Tell the police exactly what you remember. Be honest about all your activities. Remember, nothing you did—including drinking alcohol or doing drugs—can justify rape.

Ask the hospital to take a urine (pee) sample that can be used to test for date rape drugs. The drugs leave your system quickly. Rohypnol stays in the body for several hours, and can be detected in the urine up to 72 hours after taking it. GHB leaves the body in 12 hours. Don't urinate before going to the hospital.

Don't pick up or clean up where you think the assault might have occurred. There could be evidence left behind—such as on a drinking glass or bed sheets.

Get counseling and treatment. Feelings of shame, guilt, fear, and shock are normal. A counselor can help you work through these emotions and begin the healing process. Calling a crisis center or a hotline is a good place to start. One national hotline is the National Sexual Assault Hotline at 1-800-656-HOPE.

☞ **Remember!!**

Even if a victim of sexual assault drank alcohol or willingly took drugs, the victim is NOT at fault for being assaulted. You cannot "ask for it" or cause it to happen.

Chapter 25

Alcohol And Driving: A Deadly Combination

Fatal Crashes And Fatalities Involving Alcohol-Impaired Drivers

In 2006, 13,470 people were killed in alcohol-impaired-driving crashes. These alcohol-impaired-driving fatalities accounted for 32 percent of the total motor vehicle traffic fatalities in the United States.

Traffic fatalities in alcohol-impaired-driving crashes fell by 0.8 percent, from 13,582 in 2005 to 13,470 in 2006. The 13,470 alcohol-impaired-driving fatalities in 2006 were almost the same as compared to 13,451 alcohol-impaired-driving fatalities reported in 1996.

Drivers are considered to be alcohol-impaired when their blood alcohol concentration (BAC) is .08 grams per deciliter (g/dL) or higher. Thus, any fatality occurring in a crash involving a driver with a BAC of .08 or higher is considered to be an alcohol-impaired-driving fatality. The term "driver" refers to the operator of any motor vehicle, including a motorcycle.

Estimates of alcohol-impaired driving are generated using BAC values reported to the Fatality Analysis Reporting System (FARS) and imputed

About This Chapter: This chapter begins with information excerpted from "Alcohol-Impaired Driving," DOT HS 810 801, National Highway Traffic Safety Administration, March 2008. Text under the heading "Preventing Impaired Driving" is excerpted from "Impaired Driving," Centers for Disease Control and Prevention (CDC), June 2008.

Table 25.1. Fatalities, by Role, in Crashes Involving at Least One Driver With a BAC of .08 or Higher, 2006.

Role	Number	Percent Of Total
Driver With BAC = .08+	8,615	64.0%
Passenger Riding w/Driver With BAC = .08+	2,429	18.0%
Subtotal	**11,044**	**82.0%**
Occupants Of Other Vehicles	1,601	11.9%
Nonoccupants	825	6.1%
Total Fatalities	**13,470**	**100.0%**

BAC values when they are not reported. The term "alcohol-impaired" does not indicate that a crash or a fatality was caused by alcohol impairment.

The 13,470 fatalities in alcohol-impaired-driving crashes during 2006 represent an average of one alcohol-impaired-driving fatality every 39 minutes. In 2006, all 50 States, the District of Columbia, and Puerto Rico had by law created a threshold making it illegal per se to drive with a BAC of .08 or higher. Of the 13,470 people who died in alcohol-impaired-driving crashes in 2006, 8,615 (64%) were drivers with a BAC of .08 or higher. The remaining fatalities consisted of 4,030 (30%) motor vehicle occupants and 825 (6%) nonoccupants.

The national rate of alcohol-impaired-driving fatalities in motor vehicle crashes in 2006 was 0.45 per 100 million vehicle miles of travel.

Children

In 2006, 1,794 children age 14 and younger were killed in motor vehicle crashes. Of those 1,794 fatalities, 306 (17%) occurred in alcohol-impaired driving crashes. Children riding in vehicles with drivers who had a BAC level of .08 or higher accounted for half (153) of these deaths.

Another 45 children age 14 and younger who were killed in traffic crashes in 2006, were pedestrians or pedalcyclists who were struck by drivers with a BAC of .08 or higher.

Time Of Day And Day Of Week

The rate of alcohol impairment among drivers involved in fatal crashes was four times higher at night than during the day (36% versus 9%). In 2006, 15 percent of all drivers involved in fatal crashes during the week were alcohol-impaired, compared to 31 percent on weekends.

Table 25.2. Drivers in Fatal Crashes with a BAC of .08 or Higher, by Time of Day and Day of Week, 1996 and 2006.

Drivers Involved in Fatal Crashes	Total Drivers						Change in Percentage with BAC .08 or Higher 1996-2006
	1996			2006			
	Total Number of Drivers	BAC .08 or Higher		Total Number of Drivers	BAC .08 or Higher		
		Number	Percent of Total		Number	Percent of Total	
Total	57,001	12,348	22%	57,695	12,491	22%	0%
Drivers by Crash Type and Time of Day							
Single-Vehicle Crash							
Total	21,021	7,834	37%	22,627	8,391	37%	0%
Daytime*	8,019	1,366	17%	8,811	1,560	18%	+6%
Nighttime**	12,699	6,285	49%	13,525	6,672	49%	0%
Multiple Vehicle Crash							
Total	35,980	4,514	13%	35,068	4,100	12%	-8%
Daytime*	22,783	1,240	5%	21,690	1,102	5%	0%
Nighttime**	13,165	3,266	25%	13,334	2,990	22%	-12%
Drivers by Time of Day							
Daytime*	30,802	2,606	8%	30,501	2,662	9%	+13%
Nighttime**	25,864	9,552	37%	26,859	9,662	36%	-3%
Drivers by Day of Week and Time of Day							
Weekday***	34,973	5,268	15%	34,363	5,218	15%	0%
Daytime*	22,916	1,512	7%	22,030	1,469	7%	0%
Nighttime**	11,953	3,703	31%	12,223	3,702	30%	-3%
Weekend****	21,921	7,025	32%	23,240	7,234	31%	-3%
Daytime*	7,886	1,094	14%	8,471	1,193	14%	0%
Nighttime**	13,911	5,848	42%	14,636	5,960	41%	-2%

*6 a.m. to 6 p.m. **6 p.m. to 6 a.m. ***Monday 6 a.m. to Friday 6 p.m.

****Friday 6 p.m. to Monday 6 a.m.

Drivers

In fatal crashes in 2006, the highest percentage of drivers with a BAC level of .08 or higher was for drivers ages 21–24 (33%), followed by ages 25–34 (29%) and 35-44 (25%).

The percentages of drivers involved in fatal crashes with a BAC level of .08 or higher in 2006 were 27 percent for motorcycle operators, 24 percent for light trucks, and 23 percent for passenger cars. The percentage of drivers with BAC levels of .08 or higher in fatal crashes was the lowest for large trucks (1%).

♣ It's A Fact!!
Groups At Risk

- Male drivers involved in fatal motor vehicle crashes are almost twice as likely as female drivers to be intoxicated with a blood alcohol concentration (BAC) of 0.08% or greater. It is illegal to drive with a BAC of 0.08% or higher in all 50 states, the District of Columbia, and Puerto Rico.

- At all levels of blood alcohol concentration, the risk of being involved in a crash is greater for young people than for older people. In 2005, 16% of drivers ages 16 to 20 who died in motor vehicle crashes had been drinking alcohol.

- Young men ages 18 to 20 (under the legal drinking age) reported driving while impaired more frequently than any other age group.

- Among motorcycle drivers killed in fatal crashes, 30% have BACs of 0.08% or greater.

- Nearly half of the alcohol-impaired motorcyclists killed each year are age 40 or older, and motorcyclists ages 40 to 44 years have the highest percentage of fatalities with BACs of 0.08% or greater.

- Of the 1,946 traffic fatalities among children ages zero to 14 years in 2005, 21% involved alcohol.

- Among drivers involved in fatal crashes, those with BAC levels of 0.08% or higher were nine times more likely to have a prior conviction for driving while impaired (DWI) than were drivers who had not consumed alcohol.

Source: CDC, June 2008.

Seat belts were used by only 26 percent of fatally injured drivers with BAC levels of .08 or higher, compared to 39 percent of fatally injured drivers with BAC levels between .01 and .07, and 57 percent of fatally injured drivers with no alcohol (BAC = .00).

Drivers with a BAC level of .08 or higher involved in fatal crashes were eight times more likely to have a prior conviction for driving while impaired (DWI) than were drivers with no alcohol (8% and 1%, respectively).

In 2006, 84 percent (12,491) of the 14,840 drivers with a BAC of .01 or higher who were involved in fatal crashes had BAC levels at or above .08, and 55 percent (8,201) had BAC levels at or above .15. The most frequently recorded BAC level among drinking drivers in fatal crashes was .16.

Table 25.3. Drivers in Fatal Crashes with a BAC of .08 or Higher, by Age, Gender, and Vehicle Type, 1996 and 2006.

	Total Drivers					
	1996			**2006**		Change in
		BAC .08 or Higher			BAC .08 or Higher	Percentage with BAC .08
Drivers Involved in Fatal Crashes	Total Number of Drivers	Number	Percent of Total	Total Number of Drivers	Number	Percent of Total	or Higher 1996-2006
Total	57,001	12,348	22%	57,695	12,491	22%	0%
Drivers by Age Group (Years)						
16-20	7,824	1,359	17%	7,286	1,350	19%	+12%
21-24	6,205	1,950	31%	6,454	2,145	33%	+6%
25-34	12,889	3,837	30%	11,223	3,259	29%	-3%
35-44	10,955	2,765	25%	10,310	2,595	25%	0%
45-54	7,127	1,272	18%	9,201	1,746	19%	+6%
55-64	4,237	512	12%	5,864	753	13%	+8%
65-74	3,319	275	8%	3,022	229	8%	0%
75+	3,068	145	5%	2,954	139	5%	0%
Drivers by Sex						
Male	41,376	10,240	25%	41,975	10,078	24%	-4%
Female	14,850	1,963	13%	14,655	2,168	15%	+15%
Drivers by Vehicle Type						
Passenger Cars	30,595	6,948	23%	23,988	5,430	23%	0%
Light Trucks	18,118	4,341	24%	22,185	5,255	24%	0%
Large Trucks	4,703	98	2%	4,695	69	1%	-50%
Motorcycles	2,175	768	35%	4,933	1,313	27%	-23%

Numbers shown for groups of drivers do not add to the total number of drivers due to unknown or other data not included.

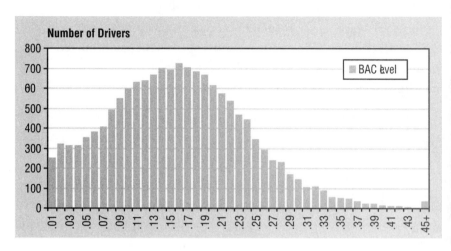

Figure 25.1. Distribution of BAC Levels for Drivers Involved in Fatal Crashes with a BAC of .01 or Higher, 2006.

Preventing Impaired Driving

Alcohol-related motor vehicle crashes kill someone every 39 minutes and injures someone non-fatally every two minutes, but there are effective measures that can be taken to prevent injuries and deaths from impaired driving.

Prevention Strategies

Effective measures to prevent injuries and deaths from impaired driving include the following:

- Aggressively enforcing existing 0.08% BAC laws, minimum legal drinking age laws, and zero tolerance laws for drivers younger than 21 years old in all states

- Promptly suspending the driver's licenses of people who drive while intoxicated

- Sobriety checkpoints

- Health promotion efforts that use an ecological framework to influence economic, organizational, policy, and school/community action

- Multi-faceted community-based approaches to alcohol control and driving-under-the-influence (DUI) prevention

- Mandatory substance abuse assessment and treatment for DUI offenders

Other measures have also been suggested to help prevent injury and death from impaired driving:

- Reducing the legal limit for blood alcohol concentration (BAC) to 0.05%

- Raising state and federal alcohol excise taxes

- Implementing compulsory blood alcohol testing when traffic crashes result in injury

Prevention Research And Evaluation

Young Drivers: Actions to decrease alcohol-related fatal crashes involving young drivers have been effective. Over the past 20 years, alcohol-related fatal crash rates have decreased by 60 percent for drivers ages 16 to 17 years and 55 percent for drivers ages 18 to 20 years, according to a study from the Centers for Disease Control and Prevention (CDC). However, this progress has stalled in the past few years. To further decrease alcohol-related fatal crashes among young drivers, communities need to implement and enforce strategies that are known to be effective, such as minimum legal drinking age laws and "zero tolerance" laws for drivers under 21 years of age.

Sobriety Checkpoints: Sobriety checkpoints reduce alcohol-related crashes. Fewer alcohol-related crashes occur when sobriety checkpoints are implemented, according to a CDC report published in the December 2002 issue of *Traffic Injury Prevention*. Sobriety checkpoints are traffic stops where law enforcement officers systematically select drivers to assess their level of alcohol impairment. The goal of these interventions is to deter alcohol-impaired driving by increasing drivers' perceived risk of arrest. The conclusion that they are effective in reducing alcohol-related crashes is based on a systematic review of research about sobriety checkpoints. The review was conducted by a team of experts led by CDC scientists, under the oversight of the Task Force on Community Preventive Services—a 15-member, non-federal group of leaders in various health-related fields. (Visit www.thecommunityguide.org for more information.) The review combined the results of 23 scientifically-sound studies from around the world. Results indicated that sobriety checkpoints consistently reduced alcohol-related crashes, typically by about 20 percent. The results were similar regardless of how the checkpoints were conducted, for short-term "blitzes," or when checkpoints were used continuously for several years. This suggests that the effectiveness of checkpoints does not diminish over time.

♣ **It's A Fact!!**

Each year, alcohol-related crashes in the United States cost about $51 billion.

Source: CDC, June 2008.

DUI Prevention Activities: Stronger state driving-under-the-influence (DUI) prevention activities may reduce alcohol-impaired driving. Strong state activities designed to prevent DUI, including legislation, enforcement, and education, may reduce the incidence of drinking and driving, according to a study from the CDC. For the study, which was published in the June 2002 issue of *Injury Prevention*, CDC analyzed data from the *1997 Behavioral Risk Factor Surveillance System (BRFSS)* national telephone survey, and the *Mothers Against Drunk Driving (MADD) Rating the States* 2000 survey, that graded states on their DUI countermeasures from 1996-1999. Results showed that residents of states with a MADD grade of "D" were 60 percent more likely to report alcohol-impaired driving than were residents from states with a MADD grade of "A." MADD based the grades on 11 categories of prevention measures, including DUI legislation; political leadership; statistics and records availability; resources devoted to enforcing DUI laws; administrative penalties and criminal sanctions; regulatory control and alcohol availability; youth DUI legislation; prevention and education; and victim compensation and support.

The study also found that four percent of the residents who consume alcohol reported they had driven after having too much to drink at least once during the previous month. Men were nearly three times as likely as women to report alcohol-impaired driving, and single people were about 50 percent more likely to report alcohol-impaired driving than married people or those living with a partner.

Effective Interventions: CDC and the Task Force on Community Preventive Services—an independent, nonfederal panel of community health experts—published systematic reviews of the literature for eight community-based interventions to reduce alcohol-impaired driving. The reviews revealed strong evidence of effectiveness for 0.08% blood alcohol concentration (BAC) laws, minimum legal drinking age laws, sobriety checkpoints, and mass media campaigns (under certain conditions). They also found sufficient evidence of effectiveness for lower BAC laws specific to young or inexperienced drivers (zero tolerance laws), school-based education programs to reduce riding with a drinking driver, and intervention training programs for alcohol servers. They found insufficient evidence of effectiveness to recommend the use of designated driver programs.

The systematic review of the effectiveness of 0.08% BAC laws for drivers was helpful in establishing a 0.08% standard nationwide. The review revealed that state laws that lowered the illegal BAC for drivers from 0.10% to 0.08% reduced alcohol-related fatalities by a median of seven percent, translating to 500 lives saved annually. With this evidence, the Task Force on Community Preventive Services strongly recommended that all states pass 0.08% BAC laws. In October 2000, the President signed the Fiscal Year 2001 transportation appropriations bill, requiring states to pass the 0.08% BAC law by October 2003 or risk losing federal highway construction funds. As of October 1, 2003, 45 states and the District of Columbia had enacted 0.08% BAC legislation.

In June 2001, Tommy G. Thompson, Secretary of the Department of Health and Human Services, awarded the Secretary's Award for Distinguished Service to the CDC researchers who conducted systematic reviews for their contribution to the field. In September 2006, Mothers Against Drunk Driving (MADD) presented the Ralph W. Hingson Research in Practice National President's Award to the CDC research team to recognize their important contributions to reducing alcohol impaired driving.

Part Four
Alcohol Abuse And Alcoholism

Chapter 26

What Is Alcoholism?

Alcoholism

Alternative Names: Alcohol dependence; alcohol abuse

Definition: Alcoholism is drinking alcoholic beverages at a level that interferes with physical health, mental health, and social, family, or job responsibilities.

Causes: Alcoholism is a type of drug addiction. There is both physical and mental dependence on alcohol.

Alcoholism is divided into two categories: dependence and abuse. People who are dependent on alcohol spend a great deal of time drinking alcohol—and getting it.

Physical dependence involves:

• A need for increasing amounts of alcohol to get drunk or achieve the desired effect (tolerance)

• Alcohol-related illnesses

About This Chapter: This chapter includes excerpts from "Alcoholism," © 2007 A.D.A.M., Inc. Reprinted with permission. Text under the heading "Frequently Asked Questions about Alcoholism," was excerpted from "FAQ for the General Public," National Institute on Alcohol Abuse and Alcoholism, February 2007.

- Memory lapses (blackouts) after drinking episodes

- Withdrawal symptoms when alcohol use is stopped

The most severe drinking behavior includes long drinking binges that lead to mental or physical problems. Some people are able to gain control over their dependence in earlier phases before they totally lose control. But no one knows which heavy drinkers will be able to regain control and which will not.

There is no known common cause of alcoholism. However, several factors may play a role in its development. A person who has an alcoholic parent is more likely to become an alcoholic than a person without alcoholism in the immediate family.

Research suggests that certain genes may increase the risk of alcoholism, but which genes or how they work is not known.

Psychological factors may include:

- A need for anxiety relief;

- Conflict in relationships;

- Depression;

- Low self-esteem.

Social factors include:

- Ease of getting alcohol;

- Peer pressure;

- Social acceptance of alcohol use;

- Stressful lifestyle.

The incidence of alcohol intake and related problems is rising. Data indicate that about 15 percent of people in the United States are problem drinkers, and about five to 10 percent of male drinkers and three to five percent of female drinkers could be diagnosed as alcohol dependent.

Symptoms: Alcohol affects the central nervous system as a depressant. This leads to a decrease in:

✎ What's It Mean?

Alcoholism: Also known as alcohol dependence, alcoholism is a disease that includes the following four symptoms:

1. **Craving:** A strong need, or urge, to drink.

2. **Loss Of Control:** Not being able to stop drinking once drinking has begun.

3. **Physical Dependence:** Withdrawal symptoms, such as nausea, sweating, shakiness, and anxiety after stopping drinking.

4. **Tolerance:** The need to drink greater amounts of alcohol to get "high."

For clinical and research purposes, formal diagnostic criteria for alcoholism also have been developed. Such criteria are included in the *Diagnostic and Statistical Manual of Mental Disorders, Fourth Edition,* published by the American Psychiatric Association, as well as in the International Classification Diseases, published by the World Health Organization.

Source: NIAAA, February 2007.

- Activity;

- Anxiety;

- Inhibitions;

- Tension.

Even a few drinks can change behavior, slow motor skills, and decrease the ability to think clearly. It can impair concentration and judgment. Drinking a lot of alcohol can cause drunkenness (intoxication).

Some of the symptoms of alcoholism include:

- Abdominal pain;

- Confusion;

- Drinking alone;

- Episodes of violence with drinking;

- Hostility when confronted about drinking;

- Lack of control over drinking—being unable to stop or reduce alcohol intake;

- Making excuses to drink;

- Nausea and vomiting;

- Need for daily or regular alcohol use to function;

- Neglecting to eat;

- Not caring for physical appearance;

- Numbness and tingling;

- Secretive behavior to hide alcohol use;

- Shaking in the morning.

Alcohol withdrawal develops because the brain adapts to the alcohol and cannot function well without the drug. Symptoms of withdrawal may include:

- Anxiety;

- Confusion or seeing and hearing things that aren't there (hallucinations);

- Death (rarely);

- Increased blood pressure;

- Loss of appetite, nausea, or vomiting;

- Psychosis;

- Raised temperature;

- Rapid heart rate;

- Restlessness or nervousness;

- Seizures;

- Tremors.

Exams And Tests: All doctors should ask their patients about their drinking. The health care provider can get a history from the family if the affected person is unwilling or unable to answer questions. A physical examination is done to identify physical problems related to alcohol use.

The following questions are used by the National Institute on Alcohol Abuse and Alcoholism to screen for alcohol abuse or dependence:

- Do you ever drive when you have been drinking?

- Do you have to drink more than before to get drunk or feel the desired effect?

♣ It's A Fact!!
What is a safe level of drinking?

People younger than age 21 should not drink at all. Other certain people should not drink at all:

- Women who are pregnant or trying to become pregnant

- People who plan to drive or engage in other activities that require alertness and skill (such as driving a car)

- People taking certain over-the-counter or prescription medications

- People with medical conditions that can be made worse by drinking

- Recovering alcoholics

For most adults, however, moderate alcohol use—up to two drinks per day for men and one drink per day for women and older people—causes few if any problems. (One drink equals one 12-ounce bottle of beer or wine cooler, one 5-ounce glass of wine, or 1.5 ounces of 80-proof distilled spirits.)

Source: NIAAA, February 2007.

- Have you felt that you should cut down on your drinking?

- Have you ever had any blackouts after drinking?

- Have you ever missed work or lost a job because of drinking?

- Is someone in your family worried about your drinking?

Outlook (Prognosis): Only 15 percent of people with alcohol dependence seek treatment for this disease. Starting drinking again after treatment is common, so it is important to maintain support systems in order to cope with any slips and ensure that they don't turn into complete reversals.

Treatment programs have varying success rates, but many people with alcohol dependency make a full recovery.

Possible complications:

- Brain degeneration;

- Cancers of the larynx, esophagus, liver, and colon;

- Cirrhosis of the liver;

- Delirium tremens (DTs);

- Depression;

- Esophageal bleeding;

- Heart muscle damage;

- High blood pressure;

- Insomnia;

- Liver disease (alcoholic hepatitis);

- Nausea, vomiting;

- Nerve damage;

- Pancreatitis;

- Poor nutrition because vitamins aren't absorbed properly;

♣ **It's A Fact!!**
Alcoholism treatment works for many people. But like other chronic illnesses, such as diabetes, high blood pressure, and asthma, there are varying levels of success when it comes to treatment. Some people stop drinking and remain sober. Others have long periods of sobriety with bouts of relapse. And still others cannot stop drinking for any length of time. With treatment, one thing is clear, however: the longer a person abstains from alcohol, the more likely he or she will be able to stay sober.

Source: NIAAA, February 2007.

• Problems getting an erection in men;

• Severe memory loss;

• Stopping of the period (menstruation) in women;

• Suicide;

• Wernicke-Korsakoff syndrome.

Alcohol consumption during pregnancy can cause severe birth defects. The most serious is fetal alcohol syndrome, which may lead to mental retardation and behavior problems. A milder form of the condition that can still cause lifelong problems is called fetal alcohol affects.

People who are dependent on or who abuse alcohol continue to drink it despite physical or mental problems. They may have problems with binge drinking (drinking six or more drinks at one sitting). Those with dependence have more severe problems and a greater need to drink.

Alcoholism is a major social, economic, and public health problem. Alcohol is involved in more than half of all accidental deaths and almost half of all traffic deaths. A high percentage of suicides involve the use of alcohol along with other substances.

People who abuse or are dependent on alcohol are more likely to be unemployed, involved in domestic violence, and have problems with the law (such as drinking and driving).

Frequently Asked Questions About Alcoholism

Is alcoholism a disease?

Yes, alcoholism is a disease. The craving that an alcoholic feels for alcohol can be as strong as the need for food or water. An alcoholic will continue to drink despite serious family, health, or legal problems.

Like many other diseases, alcoholism is chronic, meaning that it lasts a person's lifetime; it usually follows a predictable course; and it has symptoms. The risk for developing alcoholism is influenced both by a person's genes and by his or her lifestyle.

Is alcoholism inherited?

Research shows that the risk for developing alcoholism does indeed run in families. The genes a person inherits partially explain this pattern, but lifestyle is also a factor. Currently, researchers are working to discover the actual genes that put people at risk for alcoholism. Your friends, the amount of stress in your life, and how readily available alcohol is also are factors that may increase your risk for alcoholism.

☞ Remember!!

Risk is not destiny. Just because alcoholism tends to run in families doesn't mean that a child of an alcoholic parent will automatically become an alcoholic too. Some people develop alcoholism even though no one in their family has a drinking problem. By the same token, not all children of alcoholic families get into trouble with alcohol. Knowing you are at risk is important, though, because then you can take steps to protect yourself from developing problems with alcohol.

Source: NIAAA, February 2007.

Can alcoholism be cured?

No, alcoholism cannot be cured at this time. Even if an alcoholic hasn't been drinking for a long time, he or she can still suffer a relapse. Not drinking is the safest course for most people with alcoholism.

Can alcoholism be treated?

Yes, alcoholism can be treated. Alcoholism treatment programs use both counseling and medications to help a person stop drinking. Treatment has helped many people stop drinking and rebuild their lives.

Which medications treat alcoholism?

Three oral medications—disulfiram (Antabuse®), naltrexone (Depade®, ReVia®), and acamprosate (Campral®)—are currently approved to treat alcohol dependence. In addition, an injectable, long-acting form of naltrexone (Vivitrol®) is available. These medications have been shown to help people with dependence reduce their drinking, avoid relapse to heavy drinking, and achieve and maintain abstinence. Naltrexone acts in the brain to reduce craving for alcohol after someone has stopped drinking. Acamprosate is thought to work by reducing symptoms that follow lengthy abstinence, such as anxiety and insomnia. Disulfiram discourages drinking by making the person taking it feel sick after drinking alcohol.

Other types of drugs are available to help manage symptoms of withdrawal (such as shakiness, nausea, and sweating) if they occur after someone with alcohol dependence stops drinking.

Although medications are available to help treat alcoholism, there is no "magic bullet." In other words, no single medication is available that works in every case and/or in every person. Developing new and more effective medications to treat alcoholism remains a high priority for researchers.

Do you have to be an alcoholic to experience problems?

No. Alcoholism is only one type of an alcohol problem. Alcohol abuse can be just as harmful. A person can abuse alcohol without actually being an alcoholic—that is, he or she may drink too much and too often but still not be dependent on alcohol. Some of the problems linked to alcohol abuse include not being able to meet work, school, or family responsibilities; drunk-driving arrests and car crashes; and drinking-related medical conditions. Under some circumstances, even social or moderate drinking is dangerous— for example, when driving, during pregnancy, or when taking certain medications.

Are specific groups of people more likely to have problems?

Alcohol abuse and alcoholism cut across gender, race, and nationality. In the United States, 17.6 million people—about one in every 12 adults—abuse alcohol or are alcohol dependent. In general, more men than women are alcohol dependent or have alcohol problems. And alcohol problems are highest among young adults ages 18–29 and lowest among adults ages 65 and older. We also know that people who start drinking at an early age—for example, at age 14 or younger—are at much higher risk of developing alcohol problems at some point in their lives compared to someone who starts drinking at age 21 or after.

How can you tell if someone has a problem?

Answering the following four questions can help you find out if you or a loved one has a drinking problem:

• Have you ever felt you should cut down on your drinking?

• Have people annoyed you by criticizing your drinking?

• Have you ever felt bad or guilty about your drinking?

• Have you ever had a drink first thing in the morning to steady your nerves or to get rid of a hangover?

One "yes" answer suggests a possible alcohol problem. More than one "yes" answer means it is highly likely that a problem exists. If you think that you or someone you know might have an alcohol problem, it is important to see a doctor or other health care provider right away. They can help you determine if a drinking problem exists and plan the best course of action.

Can a problem drinker simply cut down?

It depends. If that person has been diagnosed as an alcoholic, the answer is "no." Alcoholics who try to cut down on drinking rarely succeed. Cutting out alcohol—that is, abstaining—is usually the best course for recovery. People who are not alcohol dependent but who have experienced alcohol-related problems may be able to limit the amount they drink. If they can't stay within those limits, they need to stop drinking altogether.

If an alcoholic is unwilling to get help, what can you do about it?

This can be a challenge. An alcoholic can't be forced to get help except under certain circumstances, such as a traffic violation or arrest that results in court-ordered treatment. But you don't have to wait for someone to "hit rock bottom" to act. Many alcoholism treatment specialists suggest the following steps to help an alcoholic get treatment:

- Stop all "cover ups." Family members often make excuses to others or try to protect the alcoholic from the results of his or her drinking. It is important to stop covering for the alcoholic so that he or she experiences the full consequences of drinking.

- Time your intervention. The best time to talk to the drinker is shortly after an alcohol-related problem has occurred—like a serious family argument or an accident. Choose a time when he or she is sober, both of you are fairly calm, and you have a chance to talk in private.

- Be specific. Tell the family member that you are worried about his or her drinking. Use examples of the ways in which the drinking has caused problems, including the most recent incident.

- State the results. Explain to the drinker what you will do if he or she doesn't go for help—not to punish the drinker, but to protect yourself from his or her problems. What you say may range from refusing to go with the person to any social activity where alcohol will be served, to moving out of the house. Do not make any threats you are not prepared to carry out.

- Get help. Gather information in advance about treatment options in your community. If the person is willing to get help, call immediately for an appointment with a treatment counselor. Offer to go with the family member on the first visit to a treatment program and/or an Alcoholics Anonymous meeting.

- Call on a friend. If the family member still refuses to get help, ask a friend to talk with him or her using the steps just described. A friend who is a recovering alcoholic may be particularly persuasive, but any person who is caring and nonjudgmental may help. The intervention of more than one person, more than one time, is often necessary to coax an alcoholic to seek help.

- Find strength in numbers. With the help of a health care professional, some families join with other relatives and friends to confront an alcoholic as a group. This approach should only be tried under the guidance of a health care professional who is experienced in this kind of group intervention.

✔ **Quick Tip**

Getting Help For An Alcohol Problem

There are many national and local resources that can help. The National Drug and Alcohol Treatment Referral Routing Service provides a toll-free telephone number, 800-662-HELP (4357), offering various resource information. Through this service you can speak directly to a representative concerning substance abuse treatment, request printed material on alcohol or other drugs, or obtain local substance abuse treatment referral information in your state.

Many people also find support groups a helpful aid to recovery. The following list includes a variety of resources:

- Al-Anon/Alateen: http://www.al-anon.alateen.org

- Alcoholics Anonymous (AA): http://www.alcoholics-anonymous.org

- National Association for Children of Alcoholics (NACOA): http://www.nacoa.org

- National Clearinghouse for Alcohol and Drug Information (NCADI): http://www.health.org

Source: NIAAA, February 2007.

- Get support. It is important to remember that you are not alone. Support groups offered in most communities include Al-Anon, which holds regular meetings for spouses and other significant adults in an alcoholic's life, and Alateen, which is geared to children of alcoholics. These groups help family members understand that they are not responsible for an alcoholic's drinking and that they need to take steps to take care of themselves, regardless of whether the alcoholic family member chooses to get help.

You can call the National Drug and Alcohol Treatment Referral Routing Service (Center for Substance Abuse Treatment) at 800-662-HELP (4357) for information about treatment programs in your local community and to speak to someone about an alcohol problem.

Chapter 27

What Causes Alcoholism?

People have been drinking alcohol for about 15,000 years. Drinking steadily and consistently over time can produce dependence and cause withdrawal symptoms during periods of abstinence. This physical dependence, however, is not the sole cause of alcoholism. To develop alcoholism, other factors usually come into play, including biology, genetics, culture, and psychology.

Genetic Factors

Genetic factors play a significant role in alcoholism and may account for about half of the total risk for alcoholism. The role that genetics plays in alcoholism is complex, however, and it is likely that many different genes are involved. Research suggests that alcohol dependence, and other substance addictions, may be associated with genetic variations in 51 different chromosomal regions.

Researchers are investigating a number of inherited traits that make particular individuals susceptible to this disorder:

- The amygdala is an area of the brain thought to play a role in the emotional aspects of craving, which can lead to addiction. Some studies indicate that the amygdala is smaller in subjects with family histories of alcoholism, suggesting that inherited differences in brain structure may affect risk. Other studies suggest that certain brain chemicals (neurotransmitters) and proteins in the amygdala region may be involved in the link between anxiety and alcoholism.

• Some studies indicate that people may inherit a lack of the warning signals that ordinarily make people stop drinking. Research suggests this factor may contribute to 40–60% of alcoholism cases related to genetic factors. (Even in the absence of genetic factors, repeated exposure to alcohol increases the ability to tolerate larger amounts before experiencing behavioral impairment.)

• Some people with alcoholism may have an inherited dysfunction in the transmission of serotonin. Serotonin is a brain chemical messenger (neurotransmitter). It is important for well-being and associated behaviors (eating, relaxation, and sleep). Abnormal serotonin levels are associated with high levels of tolerance for alcohol. They are also linked to impulsivity and aggressiveness. These behaviors can predispose people to drink and can increase the risk for dangerous behaviors and suicide in people who are alcohol dependent.

• Dopamine is another neurotransmitter associated with alcoholism and other addictions. Research indicates that high levels of the D2 dopamine receptor may help inhibit behavioral responses to alcohol, and protect against alcoholism, in people with a family history of alcohol dependence.

Even if genetic factors can be identified, however, they are unlikely to explain all cases of alcoholism. Inheriting genetic traits does not doom a child to an alcoholic future. Environment, personality, and emotional factors also play a strong role.

Brain Chemical Imbalances After Long-Term Alcohol Use

Alcohol has widespread effects on the brain and can affect neurons (nerve cells), brain chemistry, and blood flow within the frontal lobes of the brain. Researchers are particularly interested in systems of neurotransmitters (chemical messengers) in the brain that are affected by alcohol. Some research is focusing on the way these neurotransmitters are employed in the brain after long-term alcohol use in order to adapt to the cravings and pain of withdrawal. Such chemical changes may lead to dependency or to relapse after quitting in two ways:

• They increase the need to reduce agitation

• They increase the desire to restore pleasurable feelings

When a person who is dependent on alcohol stops drinking, chemical responses create an overexcited nervous system and agitation by changing the level of chemicals that inhibit impulsivity or stress and excitation. High norepinephrine levels, a chemical the brain produces more of when drinking is stopped, in fact, may be the primary factor in withdrawal symptoms, such as an increase in blood pressure and heart rate. This hyperactivity in the brain produces an intense need to calm down and to use more alcohol. One study suggested that the need to relieve agitation may be the more important factor in causing a relapse than restoring mood.

Drinking alcohol stimulates the release of neurotransmitters (serotonin, dopamine, and opioid peptides) that produce pleasurable feelings such as euphoria, a sensation of being rewarded, and a sense of well-being.

Over time, however, heavy alcohol use appears to deplete the stores of dopamine and serotonin. Persistent drinking, therefore, eventually fails to restore mood, but by then the drinker has been conditioned to believe that alcohol will improve spirits (even though it does not).

Risk Factors

About 90% of adults in the U.S. drink alcohol. Every day, more than 700,000 Americans are being treated for alcoholism. In addition, up to half of American men have problems that are caused by alcohol.

Age

Drinking In Adolescence: About half of under-age Americans have used alcohol. About two million people ages 12–20 are considered heavy drinkers, and 4.4 million are binge drinkers. Anyone who begins drinking in adolescence is at risk for developing alcoholism. The earlier a person begins drinking, the greater the risk. A 2006 survey of over 40,000 adults indicated that among those who began drinking before age 14, nearly half had become alcoholic dependent by the age of 21. In contrast, only 9% of people who began drinking after the age of 21 developed alcoholism.

Young people at highest risk for early drinking are those with a history of abuse, family violence, depression, and stressful life events. People with a family history of alcoholism are also more likely to begin drinking before the age of 20 and to become alcoholic. Such adolescent drinkers are also more apt to underestimate the effects of drinking and to make judgment errors, such as going on binges or driving after drinking, than young drinkers without a family history of alcoholism.

> ✤ **It's A Fact!!**
>
> It is important to understand that whether they inherit the disorder or not, people with alcoholism are still legally responsible for their actions.

Drinking In The Elderly Population: Although alcoholism usually develops in early adulthood, the elderly are not exempt. In fact, doctors may overlook alcoholism when evaluating elderly patients, mistakenly attributing the signs of alcohol abuse to the normal effects of the aging process. A survey of adults over 60 reported that 15% of men and 12% of women were hazardous drinkers, and 9% of men and 3% of women were alcohol dependent.

Alcohol also affects the older body differently. People who maintain the same drinking patterns as they age can easily develop alcohol dependency without realizing it. It takes fewer drinks to become intoxicated, and older organs can be damaged by smaller amounts of alcohol than those of younger people. Also, up to one-half of the 100 most prescribed drugs for older people react adversely with alcohol. Medications used for arthritis or pain pose a particular danger for interaction with alcohol.

Gender: Most alcoholics are men, but the incidence of alcoholism in women has been increasing over the past 30 years. Studies indicate that about 7% of men and 2.5% of women abuse alcohol. However, studies suggest that women are more vulnerable than men to many of the long-term consequences of alcoholism. For example, women are more likely than men to develop alcoholic hepatitis and to die from cirrhosis, and women are more vulnerable to the brain cell damage caused by alcohol.

History Of Abuse: Individuals who were abused as children have a higher risk for substance abuse later on. In one study, 72% of women and 27% of men with substance abuse disorders reported physical or sexual abuse or both. They also had worse response to treatment than those without such a history.

Psychiatric And Behavioral Disorders

Psychiatric Disorders: Severely depressed or anxious people are at high risk for alcoholism, smoking, and other forms of addiction. Likewise, a large proportion of alcohol-dependent people suffer from an accompanying psychiatric or substance abuse disorder. Either anxiety or depression may increase the risk for self-medication with alcohol. Depression is the most common psychiatric problem in people with alcoholism or substance abuse.

Depression is less reported in the male population, but this may be caused by a male tendency to mask emotional disorders with behavior such as alcohol abuse.

Specific anxiety disorders, such as panic disorders and social phobia, may pose particular risks for alcohol and substance abuse. Social phobia causes an intense fear of being publicly scrutinized and humiliated. Panic disorders

♣ It's A Fact!!
Ethnicity: Overall, there is no difference in alcoholic prevalence among African-Americans, Caucasians, and Hispanic-Americans. Some population groups, however, such as Native Americans, have an increased incidence of alcoholism while others, such as Jewish and Asian Americans, have a lower risk. Although the biological or cultural causes of such different risks are not known, certain people in these population groups may have a genetic susceptibility or invulnerability to alcoholism because of the way they metabolize alcohol.

cause intense anxiety and panic attacks. People with these disorders may use alcohol as a way to become less inhibited in public situations or to calm feelings of panic. While anxiety disorders are found in about 15% of adults overall, over 50% of people with alcohol abuse problems suffer from these conditions. People who have anxiety disorders are more likely to resume drinking after treatment for alcohol dependence.

Long-term alcoholism itself may cause chemical changes that produce anxiety and depression. In fact, a study on elderly people with depression reported that when even moderate drinkers reduced consumption, their mood improved. Studies also indicate that alcohol use may promote panic attacks. It is not always clear, then, whether people with emotional disorders are self-medicating with alcohol, or whether alcohol itself is producing mood swings.

Behavioral Disorders And Lack of Impulse Control: Studies are also finding that alcoholism is strongly related to impulsive, excitable, and novelty-seeking behavior, and such patterns are established early on. Children who later become alcoholics or who abuse drugs are more likely to have less fear of new situations than others, even if there is a greater risk for harm than in nonalcoholics. Specifically, children with attention deficit hyperactivity disorder (ADHD), a condition that shares these behaviors, have a higher risk for alcoholism in adulthood. The risk is especially high in children with ADHD and conduct disorder.

Socioeconomic Factors: Alcoholism is not restricted to any social or economic levels. For example, a thorough 1996 study reported no higher prevalence of alcoholism among adult welfare recipients than in the general population (about 7%). There was also no difference in prevalence between African-Americans and Caucasians in low-income groups. On the other hand, people in low-income groups who drank did display some tendencies that differed from the general population of drinkers. For instance, in one study as many women as men were heavy drinkers in lower income groups. Excessive drinking may also be more dangerous in lower income groups. One study found that alcohol was a major factor in the higher death rate of people, particularly men, in lower socioeconomic groups compared with those in higher groups.

Chapter 28

What Are The Signs Of An Alcohol Problem?

Alcohol Use And Dependence

Moderate alcohol use by adults is normal, but alcohol abuse or dependence is a serious problem. Too much alcohol affects the central nervous system and how the brain functions. It affects perception, thinking, and co-ordination. It impairs judgment, reduces inhibitions, and increases aggression. Those who abuse alcohol are more likely than others to engage in high risk, thoughtless, or violent behaviors.

Abuse Vs. Dependence

Alcoholism is a term commonly used to describe the medical disorder of alcohol dependence. Many health professionals prefer more precise language that distinguishes between alcohol dependence and alcohol abuse.

Alcohol dependence is an illness with four main features:

• Physical dependence, with a characteristic withdrawal syndrome that is relieved by more alcohol (for example, morning drinking) or other drugs

About This Chapter: This chapter includes excerpts from "Alcohol Abuse And Dependence," an undated document produced by the U.S. Department of Agriculture. The text is available online at http://www.da.usda.gov/pdsd/Security%20Guide/Eap/Alcohol.htm; accessed October 2008.

- Physiological tolerance, so that more and more alcohol is needed to produce the desired effects

- Difficulty in controlling how much alcohol is consumed once drinking has begun

- A craving for alcohol that can lead to relapse if one tries to abstain

Alcohol abuse is different from alcohol dependence. Abusers are not necessarily physically addicted to alcohol, but develop problems as a result of

♣ **It's A Fact!!**
What Are The Signs Of Addiction To Alcohol?

Alcoholism is a disease where a person drinks too much alcohol on a regular basis and depends on alcohol to solve their problems. Even young people can have an alcohol problem. If you can relate to any of the items listed below, you should think about how alcohol is affecting your life and talk to an adult you trust for help.

- Alcohol has become more important than your schoolwork, family activities and relationships, or friendships.

- You use alcohol to escape from things that make you unhappy.

- You drink when you're mad at your parents, family, or friends.

- You can't control your drinking once you start. Even if you decide you'll only have a few drinks, you end up having a lot.

- When you drink, you act like a different person than when you are sober.

- When drinking with friends, you can drink more than anyone else.

- You have blackouts or events you don't fully remember after drinking.

Don't be afraid to talk to someone if you or someone you know has these signs. People want to help you. Talk to your parents, doctor, school counselor, or another adult you trust.

Source: Excerpted from "Straight Talk about Alcohol: What Are the Signs of Addiction to Alcohol?" National Women's Health Information Center (NWHIC), March 2008.

their alcohol consumption and poor judgment, failure to understand the risks, or lack of concern about damage to themselves or others. Because they are not addicted, alcohol abusers remain in control of their behavior and can change their drinking patterns in response to explanations and warnings. There are two signs of an alcohol abuser:

- Persists in habitual drinking or occasional binge drinking that causes or exacerbates a persistent or recurrent social, school, work, financial, legal, or health problem

- Uses alcohol repeatedly under circumstances which are physically dangerous, such as driving while intoxicated

Many people who abuse alcohol eventually become alcohol dependent.

Warning Signs

The presence of any of the following indicators suggests that an individual may have a serious alcohol problem or be at high risk for developing one. Any one indicator is not conclusive evidence of a serious problem, but it is relevant circumstantial evidence and should be noted.

- Drinking is causing or exacerbating a persistent or recurring social, school, work, financial, legal, or health problem. This is the heart of the alcohol issue.

- Individual has tried unsuccessfully to cut down the extent of alcohol use. Or, once the person starts drinking, he/she sometimes loses control over the amount consumed. Both are indicators of alcohol dependence.

- Individual commonly drinks while alone. Regular solitary drinking, as compared with social drinking, indicates potential, current, or future alcohol dependence.

- Individual drinks to relax prior to social events, as compared with using alcohol at social events. Drinking prior to social events indicates potential current or future alcohol problems.

- Individual drinks first thing in the morning as an "eye-opener" or to get rid of a hangover. This is a strong indicator of dependence.

- Individual claims a high tolerance for alcohol, for example, makes statements such as: "I can drink a lot without its having any effect on me, so I don't have to worry." High tolerance is an indicator of alcohol dependence—it takes more and more to have the same effect on the body.

- Individual uses alcohol as a means of coping with life's problems. This indicates possible psychological or emotional problems and greatly increases the likelihood that alcohol already is or will become a problem. On the other hand, if motivation is experimentation, peer pressure, or adolescent rebelliousness, this does not necessarily predict future abuse.

- There has been a recent increase in individual's drinking. A change for the worse in drinking pattern may signal the existence of other relevant issues.

🖝 Remember!!

When people drink too much, with time they risk becoming addicted to alcohol. This is called alcoholism, or alcohol dependence. It's a disease, and it can happen at any age. Common signs include the ones listed below.

- **Craving:** A strong need or urge to drink

- **Loss Of Control:** Not being able to stop or cut down drinking

- **Not Feeling Well After Heavy Drinking:** Upset stomach, sweating, shakiness, or nervousness

- **A Need To Drink More:** To get the same effect as before

- **Neglecting Activities:** Giving up or cutting back on other activities

- **Continuing To Drink:** Even though alcohol is causing problems

It may be hard to imagine why people with alcoholism can't just "use a little willpower" to stop drinking. But the addiction creates an uncontrollable need for alcohol. It can be as strong as the need for food and water. People may want to stop because they know that drinking harms their health and their loved ones. But quitting is extremely difficult.

Although some people are able to recover from alcoholism without help, many need assistance. With treatment and support, many stop drinking and rebuild their lives.

Source: "Too Much, Too Soon, Too Risky," National Institute on Alcohol Abuse and Alcoholism (http://www.thecoolspot.gov), 2004.

- There is a family history of alcohol abuse. Genetic studies indicate that alcoholism tends to run in families and that a genetic vulnerability to alcoholism exists. The disruption of family life in an alcoholic home also plays a role in creating vulnerability to alcoholism later in life. On the other hand, many children react to parental alcoholism by carefully avoiding alcohol themselves. According to one study, the chances the child will follow in the parent's footsteps depend, in part, upon which parent is the alcoholic and the nature of the relationship with that parent. Children of alcoholic mothers are at far greater risk than children of alcoholic fathers.

Getting Beyond Denial

Most alcohol abusers and alcoholics deny they have a problem. As they develop dependence on alcohol, they also develop "blinders"—a defense system that allows them to ignore the problem. They want to blame their problems on something or someone else—bad luck, a misunderstanding parent, a teacher who doesn't like them, etc.

Recognizing and accepting that an alcohol problem exists is the first, crucial step toward solving the problem. If you have an alcohol problem, it is important to keep the following in mind. If you are concerned about a family member or friend who has a problem, share these thoughts with that person.

- Alcoholism is an illness, not a moral weakness. Blaming yourself, blaming others, or feeling ashamed about your drinking are all stumbling blocks to receiving help.

- You are not alone. The National Institute on Alcohol Abuse and Alcoholism estimates 14 million Americans—one of every 13 adults—either abuse alcohol or are alcoholics. Each year about 600,000 patients enter treatment for alcoholism.

- Don't push away the messengers. People who worry or complain about your drinking can be a key to your recovery. They care enough about you to be concerned. If you are an alcoholic, you'll need their support.

- The earlier the treatment, the more successful it is likely to be. Don't wait until the health effects are irreversible, you have failed in school, or your family life has suffered.

- Heavy drinking has serious health consequences. It increases the risk of cancer and causes liver damage, immune system problems, brain damage and harm to the fetus during pregnancy. It also increases the risk of accidents and mental problems.

Chapter 29

Recognizing And Diagnosing Alcoholism

Alcohol Abuse: How To Recognize Problem Drinking

[Editor's Note: Although the text in this section describes problem drinking and heavy drinking in adults; teens—who should not drink at all—may still find these facts informative.]

Am I drinking too much?

Yes, if you are:

- A woman who has more than seven drinks* per week or more than three drinks per occasion;

- A man who has more than 14 drinks* per week or more than four drinks per occasion; or

- Older than 65 years and having more than seven drinks* per week or more than three drinks per occasion.

*One drink equals one 12-ounce bottle of beer (4.5 percent alcohol), one 5-ounce glass of wine (12.9 percent alcohol), or 1.5 ounces of 80-proof distilled spirits.

Am I drinking heavily?

Yes, if you are:

- A woman who has more than three drinks every day or 21 drinks per week; or

- A man who has more than five drinks every day or 35 drinks per week.

Am I taking risks with alcohol?

Yes, if you:

- Drink and drive, operate machinery, or mix alcohol with medicine (over-the-counter and prescription medicine);

- Don't tell your surgeon, physician, or pharmacist that you are a regular drinker;

- Are pregnant or are trying to become pregnant and drink at all (even small amounts of alcohol may hurt an unborn child); or

- Drink alcohol while you are looking after small children.

Has my drinking become a habit?

Yes, if you drink regularly to:

- Relax, relieve anxiety, or go to sleep;

- Be more comfortable in social situations;

- Avoid thinking about sad or unpleasant things; or

- Socialize with other regular drinkers.

Is alcohol taking over my life?

Yes, if you:

- Ever worry about having enough alcohol for an evening or weekend;

- Hide alcohol or buy it at different stores so people will not know how much you are drinking;

- Switch from one kind of drink to another hoping that this will keep you from drinking too much or getting drunk; or

- Try to get "extra" drinks at a social event or sneak drinks when others aren't looking.

Has drinking alcohol become a problem for me?

Yes, if you:

- Can't stop drinking once you start;

- Have tried to stop drinking for a week or so but only quit for a few days;

- Fail to do what you should at work or at home because of drinking;

- Feel guilty after drinking;

- Find other people make comments to you about your drinking;

- Have a drink in the morning to get yourself going after drinking heavily the night before;

- Can't remember what happened while you were drinking; or

- Have hurt someone else as a result of your drinking.

What can I do about drinking too much?

Try to cut down to safe drinking levels: less than seven drinks per week and less than three drinks per occasion for women and older people, and less than 14 drinks per week and less than four drinks per occasion for men.

How can I get help for an alcohol problem?

If you feel you need help to cut down, you can contact:

- Your doctor for advice, treatment, or referral;

- Self-help support groups; or

- Center for Substance Abuse Treatment (800-662-HELP). Call for information about local treatment programs and to speak to someone about your alcohol problem.

Diagnostic Tools For Alcoholism

Even when people with alcoholism experience withdrawal symptoms, they nearly always deny the problem, leaving it up to co-workers, friends, or relatives to recognize the symptoms and to take the first steps toward encouraging treatment. Denial, in fact, may be an important warning signal for alcoholism.

Family members cannot always rely on a doctor to make an initial diagnosis. Although 15–30% of people who are hospitalized have alcoholism or alcohol dependence, doctors often fail to screen for the problem. In addition, doctors themselves often do not recognize the symptoms. Even when doctors identify an alcohol problem, however, they are frequently reluctant to confront the patient with a diagnosis that might lead to treatment for addiction.

Screening Tests For Alcoholism

A number of short screening tests are available, which a person can even take on their own. Because people with alcoholism often deny their problem or otherwise attempt to hide it, the tests are designed to elicit answers related to problems associated with drinking rather than the amount of liquor consumed or other specific drinking habits.

♣ It's A Fact!!

Laboratory Tests: Tests for alcohol levels in the blood are not useful for diagnosing alcoholism because they reflect consumption at only one point in time and not long-term usage. Certain blood tests, however, may provide biologic markers that suggest medical problems associated with alcoholism or indications of alcohol abuse:

• *Carbohydrate-deficient transferrin (CDT):* This compound is a marker for heavy drinking and can be helpful in monitoring patients for progress towards abstinence.

• *Gamma-glutamyltransferase (GGT):* This liver enzyme is very sensitive to alcohol and can be elevated after moderate alcohol intake and in chronic alcoholism.

• *Aspartate (AST) and alanine aminotransaminases (ALT):* These are liver enzymes and are markers for liver damage.

• *Testosterone:* Male hormone levels in men with alcoholism may be low. (Such results sometimes persuade men with alcoholism to seek help.)

• *Mean corpuscular volume (MCV):* This blood test measures the size of red blood cells, which increase with alcohol use over time.

Source: © 2007 A.D.A.M., Inc. Reprinted with permission.

CAGE Test: The CAGE test is an acronym for the following questions and is the quickest test:

- Attempts to CUT (C) down on drinking

- ANNOYANCE (A) with criticisms about drinking

- GUILT (G) about drinking

- Use of alcohol as an EYE-OPENER (E) in the morning

This test and another called the Self-Administered Alcoholism Screening Test (SAAST) appear to be most useful in detecting possible alcoholism in white, middle-aged males. They are not very accurate for identifying alcohol abuse in older people, white women, and African-Americans and Mexican Americans.

T-ACE Test: The T-ACE test is a four-question test that appears to be quite accurate in identifying alcoholism in both men and women. It asks the following questions:

- Does it TAKE (T) more than three drinks to make you feel high?

- Have you ever been ANNOYED (A) by people's criticism of your drinking?

- Are you trying to CUT DOWN (C) on drinking?

- Have you ever used alcohol as an EYE OPENER (E) in the morning?

A positive response to two of these four questions is considered to indicate possible alcohol abuse or dependence.

AUDIT Test: A more effective and important test for most people may be the Alcohol Use Disorders Identification Test (AUDIT), which is the only test specifically designed to identify hazardous or harmful drinking. It asks three questions about amount and frequency of drinking, three questions about alcohol dependence, and four questions about problems related to alcohol consumption.

A Single-Question: One simple question may be as sensitive as the CAGE or AUDIT: "When was the last time you had more than five drinks (for men) or four drinks (for women) in one day?" An answer of "within three months" accurately identified about half of people who were problem drinkers. Problem drinking is defined as hazardous drinking within the last month or some alcohol-use disorder during the past year.

Other Screening Tests: Other short screening tests are the Michigan Alcoholism Screening Test (MAST) and the Alcohol Dependence Scale (ADS).

Chapter 30

Do I Need Help For An Alcohol Problem?

How Are Alcohol And Drugs Affecting Your Life?

Yes Or No?

1. Do you use alcohol or other drugs to build self-confidence?

2. Do you ever drink or get high immediately after you have a problem at home or at school?

3. Have you ever missed school due to alcohol or other drugs?

4. Does it bother you if someone says that you use too much alcohol or other drugs?

5. Have you started hanging out with a heavy drinking or drug using crowd?

6. Are alcohol or other drugs affecting your reputation?

7. Do you feel guilty or bummed out after using alcohol or other drugs?

8. Do you feel more at ease on a date when drinking or using other drugs?

About This Chapter: This chapter begins with "How Are Alcohol And Drugs Affecting Your Life," © 2009 National Council on Alcoholism and Drug Dependence (www.ncadd.org). All rights reserved. Reprinted with permission. Additional information from the American Academy of Family Physicians and from The Nemours Foundation is cited separately within the text.

9. Have you gotten into trouble at home for using alcohol or other drugs?

10. Do you borrow money or "do without" other things to buy alcohol and other drugs?

11. Do you feel a sense of power when you use alcohol or other drugs?

12. Have you lost friends since you started using alcohol or other drugs?

13. Do your friends use less alcohol or other drugs than you do?

14. Do you drink or use other drugs until your supply is all gone?

15. Do you ever wake up and wonder what happened the night before?

16. Have you ever been busted or hospitalized due to alcohol or use of illicit drugs?

17. Do you "turn off" any studies or lectures about alcohol or illicit drug use?

18. Do you think you have a problem with alcohol or other drugs?

19. Has there ever been someone in your family with a drinking or other drug problem?

20. Could you have a problem with alcohol or other drugs?

Purchase or public possession of alcohol is illegal for anyone under the

> ### ♣ It's A Fact!!
> ### Other Signs That Alcohol Is A Problem
>
> - Accidents
> - Anxiety
> - Being unusually suspicious
> - Blackouts/memory loss
> - Breakdown of relationships
> - Depression
> - Getting driving tickets while under the influence of alcohol
> - Insomnia
> - Loss of self-esteem
> - Not taking care of yourself
> - Poor work performance
> - Taking sick days for hangovers
> - Trembling hands
> - Trouble having erections (men)
>
> Source: Copyright © 2006 American Academy of Family Physicians. All rights Reserved.

age of 21 everywhere in the United States. Aside from the fact that you may be breaking the law by using alcohol and/or illicit drugs, if you answer "yes" to any three of the above questions, you may be at risk for developing alcoholism and/or dependence on another drug. If you answer "yes" to five of these questions, you should seek professional help immediately. Contact one of the National Council on Alcoholism and Drug Dependence affiliates who will be able to help you or call the NCAD HOPE LINE at 800-NCA-CALL using a touch tone phone.

National Council On Alcoholism And Drug Dependence (NCADD)

244 East 58th Street, 4th Floor
New York, NY 10022
Toll-Free: 800-622-2255
Phone: 212-269-7797
Fax: 212-269-7510
Website: http://www.ncadd.org
E-mail: national@ncadd.org

Alcohol: What To Do If It's A Problem For You

Reprinted with permission from "Alcohol: What To Do If It's a Problem for You," August 2006, http://familydoctor.org/online/famdocen/home/common/addictions/alcohol/006.html. Copyright © 2006 American Academy of Family Physicians. All Rights Reserved.

How can I tell if alcohol is a problem for me?

Alcohol is a problem if it causes problems in any part of your life. This includes your health, your work, and your life at home. You may have a problem with alcohol if you think about drinking all the time, if you keep trying to quit on your own but can't, or if you often drink more than you plan to.

Ask Yourself These Questions: If you answer yes to one or more of the following questions, you may have a problem with alcohol. Have you ever felt:

✔ Quick Tip

My friend thinks I have a drinking and drug problem. What should I do?

Using alcohol or drugs regularly is usually just a step away from addiction—where you depend on these substances just to feel good or get through your day.

Here are a few of the early warning signs that someone may have a substance abuse problem:

- Relying on drugs or alcohol to have fun, forget problems, or relax
- Having blackouts
- Drinking or using drugs alone
- Withdrawing or keeping secrets from friends or family
- Losing interest in activities that used to be important
- Performing differently in school (such as grades dropping and frequent absences)
- Building an increased tolerance to alcohol or drugs—gradually needing more and more of the substance to get the same feeling
- Lying, stealing, or selling stuff to get money for drugs or alcohol

It's usually hard for people to recognize they have a problem, which is why friends or family often step in. People who are addicted to drugs or alcohol may promise over and over that they'll stop. But quitting is hard to do, and many people find they can't do it without help. The best thing you can do is to talk to someone you trust—preferably an adult who can support you—so you don't have to deal with your problem alone.

Lots of resources are available for people with substance abuse problems. Alcoholics Anonymous and Narcotics Anonymous offer information and recovery programs for teens. The Alcohol and Drug Information hotline is 800-729-6686.

Source: "I Think I May Have a Drinking/Drug Problem. What Should I Do?" September 2006, reprinted with permission from www.kidshealth.org. Copyright © 2006 The Nemours Foundation. This information was provided by KidsHealth, one of the largest resources online for medically reviewed health information written for parents, kids, and teens. For more articles like this one, visit www.KidsHealth.org, or www.TeensHealth.org.

- The need to cut down on your drinking;
- Annoyed by criticism of your drinking;
- Guilty about your drinking;
- As if you need a drink in the morning?

Who has an alcohol problem?

Many people only think of a "skid-row bum" when they think of someone with an alcohol problem. This is the end stage of alcohol problems, when a person has lost his or her family, job, and health because of alcohol abuse. You don't reach this stage overnight.

You may see less obvious changes along the way, beginning with drinking more than you intended or more than is safe for what you are doing (like driving a car).

Many people find it hard to admit when alcohol is a problem. Often, people around you may see your problem before you do. Think about the things mentioned here. Think about what your friends and family say to you about drinking. Then talk with your family doctor about your concerns.

How does alcohol affect my health?

Alcohol is best known as a cause of cirrhosis, a disease of the liver. However, it has many other effects on your health. It's a major cause of deaths and injuries due to accidents. It can have severe effects on a baby during pregnancy. It can also cause stomach pain due to a bleeding ulcer or irritated stomach lining.

What causes alcoholism?

The causes of alcoholism are not fully known. A history of alcoholism in your family makes it more likely. Men seem to be more at risk than women. Some drinkers use alcohol to try to relieve anxiety, depression, tension, loneliness, self-doubt, or unhappiness.

Why should I quit?

Quitting is the only way to stop the problems alcohol is causing in your life. It may not be easy to quit, but your efforts will be rewarded with better health, better relationships, and a sense of accomplishment. As you think about quitting, you may want to make a list of your reasons to quit.

How do I stop?

The first step is realizing that you control your own behavior. It's the only real control you have in your life. So use it. Here are the next steps:

- **Commit To Quitting:** Once you decide to quit, you can make plans to be sure you succeed.

- **Get Help From Your Doctor:** He or she can be your biggest ally. Alcoholism is a kind of disease, and it can be treated. Talking with your doctor or a counselor about your problems can be helpful too.

- **Get Support:** Contact Alcoholics Anonymous or the National Council on Alcoholism and Drug Dependence. They will give you the tools and support you need to quit. Ask your family and friends for support too.

What does it feel like to quit drinking?

As you drink, your body tries to make up for the depressant effects of alcohol. This built-up tolerance to alcohol can lead to severe withdrawal symptoms when people who drink a lot quit.

Serious withdrawal symptoms include seeing things, seizures and delirium tremens (confusion, seeing vivid images, severe shakes, being very suspicious), and can even include death. This is why you may need your doctor's care if you've been drinking heavily and are trying to quit.

Chapter 31

Treating Alcoholism

Understanding Treatments For Alcoholism

Once a diagnosis of alcoholism is made, the next major step is getting the patient to seek treatment. The main reasons alcoholics do not seek treatment are:

• Lack of confidence in successful therapies;

• Denial of their own alcoholism;

• Social stigma attached to the condition and its treatment.

The alcoholic patient and everyone involved should fully understand that alcoholism is a disease. Furthermore, the responses to this disease (need, craving, fear of withdrawal) are not character flaws but symptoms, just as pain or discomfort are symptoms of other illnesses. They should also realize that treatment is difficult and sometimes painful, just as are treatments for other life-threatening diseases, such as cancer, but that treatment is the only hope for a cure.

Interventions by family members, employers, and therapists can be very effective in motivating a person to quit and in reducing drinking over the

This chapter includes excerpts from "Alcoholism," © 2007 A.D.A.M., Inc. reprinted with permission.

short term. Even brief interventions from a primary care doctor and self-help information can be helpful in reducing harmful drinking. Studies report, however, that only regular follow-up and reinforcement will sustain quit rates and possibly even improve survival rates.

Personal Intervention Meetings: The best approaches for motivating a patient to seek treatment are interventional group meetings between people with alcoholism and their friends and family members who have been affected by the alcoholic behavior. Using this approach, each person affected offers a compassionate but direct and honest report describing specifically how they have been hurt by their loved one's alcoholism. The family and friends should express their affection for the patient and their intentions for supporting the patient through recovery, but they must strongly and consistently demand that the patient seek treatment. Children may even be involved in this process, depending on their level of maturity and ability to handle the situation.

Employer Intervention: Employers can be particularly effective. Their approach should also be compassionate but strong, threatening the employee with loss of employment if they do not seek help. Some large companies provide access to inexpensive or free treatment programs for their workers. Studies suggest that such interventions are effective at helping the worker at least to cut back on drinking.

> **♣ It's A Fact!!**
>
> Individuals who become alcohol dependent before age 25 are less likely to ever seek treatment than those who become alcohol dependent at age 30 or older, according to a new study supported by the National Institute on Alcohol Abuse and Alcoholism (NIAAA), part of the National Institutes of Health (NIH). They also are more likely to have multiple dependence episodes, of longer duration, and to meet more dependence diagnostic criteria than those who become alcohol dependent later in life.
>
> Source: "Early Alcohol Dependence Linked to Reduced Treatment Seeking and Chronic Relapse," NIAAA, September 2006.

Overall Treatment Goals

The ideal goals of long-term treatment by many doctors and organizations such as Alcoholics Anonymous (AA) are total abstinence. Patients who secure total abstinence have better survival rates, mental health, and marriages, and they are more responsible parents and employees than those who continue to drink or relapse. To achieve this, the patient aims to avoid high-risk situations and replace the addictive patterns with satisfying, time-filling behaviors.

Because abstinence is so difficult to attain, however, many professionals choose to treat alcoholism as a chronic disease. In other words, patients should expect and accept relapse but should aim for as long a remission period as possible. Even merely reducing alcohol intake can lower the risk for alcohol-related medical problems.

AA and other alcoholic treatment groups are greatly worried by treatment approaches that do not aim for strict abstinence, however. Many people with alcoholism are eager for any excuse to start drinking again. There is also no way to determine which people can stop after one drink and which ones cannot. Evidence strongly suggests that seeking total abstinence and avoiding high-risk situations are the optimal goal for people with alcoholism.

Inpatient Versus Outpatient Treatment

A number of treatment options now exist for alcoholism. It is first important to determine whether inpatient or outpatient care would best benefit the individual. A variety of treatment options exist that do not require overnight stay in a hospital. Structured programs exist that involve anywhere from a couple of hours a day for several days a week to 20 or more hours per week (sometimes called partial hospitalization) of monitoring. Withdrawal and subsequent abstinence monitoring using outpatient visits to a doctor is occasionally tried for select, low-risk patients.

Inpatient care may also be performed in a general or psychiatric hospital or in a center dedicated to treatment of alcohol and other substance abuse. Factors that indicate a need for this type of treatment include:

- Coexisting medical or psychiatric disorder
- Delirium tremens
- Potential harm to selves or others
- Failure to respond to conservative treatments
- Disruptive home environment

A typical inpatient regimen may include the following stages:

- A physical and psychiatric work-up for any physical or mental disorders
- Detoxification—this phase involves initiating abstinence, managing withdrawal symptoms and complications, and ensuring that the patient remains in treatment
- On-going treatment with medications in some cases
- Psychotherapy, usually cognitive behavioral therapy
- An introduction to Alcoholics Anonymous

♣ **It's A Fact!!**
The Unique Needs Of Adolescents In Alcohol Treatment

- Adolescent alcohol use often stems from different causes than for adults. In treatment, adolescents must be approached differently from adults because of developmental issues, differences in values and belief systems, environmental considerations such as strong peer influences, and educational requirements.

- Treatment approaches should also account for age, gender, ethnicity, cultural background, family structure, cognitive and social development, and readiness for change. Younger adolescents have different developmental needs than older adolescents, and treatment approaches should be developed appropriately for different age groups.

- Treatment should involve family members because family history may play a role in the origins of the problem and successful treatment cannot take place in isolation.

- Treatment providers should have specific training in the principles of adolescent development, and treatment programs should avoid mixing adult clients with adolescent clients.

Source: "Alcohol Treatment and Adolescents," Substance Abuse and Mental Health and Human Services Administration (SAMHSA), 2000.

Some—but not all—studies have reported better success rates with inpatient treatment of patients with alcoholism. However, newer studies strongly suggest that alcoholism can be effectively treated in a doctor's office.

The new approach to outpatient treatment uses "medical management" — a disease management approach that is used for chronic illnesses such as diabetes. With medical management, patients receive regular 20-minute sessions with a health care provider. The provider monitors the patient's medical condition, medication, and alcohol consumption.

A medical management approach generally involves one or both of the following:

• Drug treatment with naltrexone (ReVia, Vivitrol)

• Behavioral counseling with a therapy technique called combined behavioral intervention (CBI)

Outpatient Treatment Options: People with mild-to-moderate withdrawal symptoms are usually treated as outpatients. Treatments are similar to those in inpatient situations and include:

• Psychotherapy or counseling;

• Medications that target brain chemicals involved in addiction;

• Social support groups such as Alcoholics Anonymous;

• Cognitive therapies;

• Quitting smoking (smoking interferes with the brain's recovery from alcoholism);

• Involvement of family and other significant people in patient's life.

After-Care And Work Therapy: After-care employs services that help alcoholics maintain sobriety. For example, in some cities, sober-living houses provide residences for people who are trying to stay sober. They do not offer formal treatment services, but the people living there offer each other support and maintain an abstinent environment. One study reported that work therapy improved the outcome for homeless veterans who were being treated for substance abuse.

Factors That Predict Success Or Failure After Treatment

About 25% of people are continuously abstinent following treatment, and another 10% use alcohol moderately and without problems. Most studies strongly suggest that intensive and prolonged treatment is important for successful recovery, whether the patient is treated within or outside a treatment center.

Certain factors play a role in success or failure. Patients from low-income groups tend to have worse results in general. Their difficulties are often intensified by lack of insurance, low self-esteem, and minimal social support.

Treating People Who Have Both Alcoholism And Health Problems

Severe alcoholism is often complicated by the presence of serious medical illnesses. People with alcoholism should try at least to maintain a healthy diet and take vitamin supplements. Such deficiencies are a major cause of health problems in people with alcoholism. Women are particularly endangered.

A program called integrated outpatient treatment (IOT) may be specifically helpful for medically ill alcoholics. The patient visits a clinic once a month and receives both intensive alcohol treatment and a physical check-up, which includes tracking factors, such as liver function, that are affected by drinking.

Treating People Who Have Both Alcoholism And Mental Illness

Treatment for patients with both alcoholism and mental illness is particularly difficult. The greater the psychiatric distress a person is experiencing, the more the person is tempted to drink, particularly in negative situations.

There has been some concern that self-help programs, such as Alcoholics Anonymous (AA), are not effective for patients with dual diagnoses of mental illness and alcoholism, because the focus of the organization is on addiction, not psychiatric problems. Studies, however, have reported that they are also effective in many of these patients. (AA may not be as helpful for people with schizophrenia and schizoaffective disorder.) In one study, individuals with a dual diagnosis achieved better abstinence rates after being treated only for alcoholism compared to patients treated for the mental disorder as well. (Cognitive-behavioral therapy was used for both groups.)

Newer antidepressants such as selective serotonin reuptake inhibitors (SSRIs) are proving to be very useful complements to AA or counseling sessions. Anti-anxiety medications are also available for people with anxiety. People with alcoholism and more severe problems such as schizophrenia or severe bipolar disorder may require other types of medications.

Treatment For Alcohol Withdrawal

When a person with alcoholism stops drinking, withdrawal symptoms begin within six to 48 hours and peak about 24–35 hours after the last drink. During this period, the inhibition of brain activity caused by alcohol is abruptly reversed. Stress hormones are overproduced, and the central nervous system becomes overexcited. Common symptoms include:

- Anxiety;

- Irritability;

- Agitation;

- Insomnia.

Additional symptoms may include:

- Extremely aggressive behavior;

- Fever;

- Rapid heartbeat;

- Changes in blood pressure (either higher or lower);

- Mental disturbances;

- Seizures occur in about 10% of adults during withdrawal. In about 60% of these patients, the seizures are multiple. The time between the first and last seizure is usually six hours or less.

- Delirium tremens (DTs) are withdrawal symptoms that become progressively severe and include altered mental states (hallucinations, confusion, severe agitation) or generalized seizures. DTs are potentially fatal. They develop in up to 5% of alcoholic patients, usually two to four days after the last drink, although it may take two or more days to peak.

It is not clear if older people with alcoholism are at higher risk for more severe symptoms than younger patients. However, several studies have indicated that they may suffer more complications during withdrawal, including delirium, falls, and a decreased ability to perform normal activities.

Initial Assessment

Upon entering a hospital due to alcohol withdrawal, patients should be given a physical examination for any injuries or medical conditions. They should be treated, if possible, for any potentially serious problems, such as high blood pressure, anemia, liver damage, or irregular heartbeat.

Treatment For Withdrawal Symptoms

The immediate goal of treatment is to calm the patient as quickly as possible. Patients should be observed for at least two hours to determine the severity of withdrawal symptoms. Doctors may use assessment tests, such as the Clinical Institute Withdrawal Assessment (CIWA) scale, to help determine treatment and whether the symptoms will progress in severity.

About 95% of people have mild-to-moderate withdrawal symptoms, including agitation, trembling, disturbed sleep, and lack of appetite. In 15–20% of people with moderate symptoms, brief seizures and hallucinations may occur, but they do not progress to full-blown delirium tremens. Such patients often can be treated as outpatients. After being examined and observed, the patient is usually sent home with a four-day supply of anti-anxiety medication, scheduled for follow-up and rehabilitation, and advised to return to the emergency room if withdrawal symptoms increase in severity. If possible, a family member or friend should support the patient through the next few days of withdrawal.

Benzodiazepines: Anti-anxiety drugs known as benzodiazepines inhibit nerve-cell excitability in the brain and are considered to be the treatment of choice. They relieve withdrawal symptoms, help prevent progression to delirium tremens, and reduce the risk for seizures. Long-acting drugs, such as chlordiazepoxide (Libritabs, Librium), oxazepam (Serax), and halazepam (Paxipam) are preferred. They pose less risk for abuse than the shorter-acting drugs, which include diazepam (Valium), alprazolam (Xanax), and lorazepam (Ativan).

Assessing symptoms frequently and administering benzodiazepine doses as needed (instead of giving to a fixed dose at regular intervals) may reduce the incidence of withdrawal symptoms and other adverse events, including delirium, seizures, and transfer to the intensive care unit.

Some doctors question the use of any anti-anxiety medication for mild withdrawal symptoms, since these drugs are subject to abuse. Others believe that repeated withdrawal episodes, even mild forms, that are inadequately treated may result in increasingly severe and frequent seizures with possible brain damage. In any case, benzodiazepines are usually not prescribed for more than two weeks or administered for more than three nights per week. Problems with benzodiazepines include:

- *Side Effects:* Common side effects of benzodiazepines are daytime drowsiness and a hung-over feeling. In rare cases, they actually cause agitation. Respiratory problems may be worsened. The drugs stimulate eating and can cause weight gain. Benzodiazepines can interact with certain drugs, including cimetidine (Tagamet), antihistamines, and oral contraceptives. Benzodiazepines are potentially dangerous when used in combination with alcohol. Overdoses are serious, although rarely fatal. Elderly people are more susceptible to side effects and should usually start at half the dose prescribed for younger people. Benzodiazepines are associated with birth defects and should not be used by pregnant women or nursing mothers.

- *Loss Of Effectiveness And Dependence:* The primary problem with these drugs is their loss of effectiveness over time with continued use at the same dosage. As a result, patients may increase their dosage level to prevent anxiety. Patients then can become dependent. In fact, some evidence suggests that people with alcoholism, or even a family history of alcoholism, may be more susceptible to benzodiazepine abuse than nonalcoholics. This is a common danger and can occur after as short a time as three months. (These drugs do not cause euphoria, a so-called "high," so such drugs are not addictive in the same way narcotics are.)

- *Withdrawal Symptoms:* People who discontinue benzodiazepines after taking them for even four weeks can experience mild rebound symptoms.

The longer the drugs are taken and the higher the dose, the more severe the symptoms. They include sleep disturbance and anxiety, which can develop within hours or days after stopping the medication. Some patients experience withdrawal symptoms, including stomach distress, sweating, and insomnia, that can last from one to three weeks. Sleep changes, in fact, can persist or months or years after quitting and may be a major factor in relapse.

Antiseizure Medications: Antiseizure drugs, such as carbamazepine (Tegretol) or divalproex sodium (Depakote), may be useful for reducing the requirements of a benzodiazepine. When used by themselves, however, they do not appear to reduce seizures or delirium associated with withdrawal.

Other Supportive Drugs: Beta-blockers, such as propranolol (Inderal) and atenolol (Tenormin), are sometimes used in combination with benzodiazepines. They slow heart rate and reduce tremors. They may also reduce cravings.

Note On Treating Alcohol Withdrawal With Alcohol: Some medical centers give patients alcohol to help with withdrawal. Experts do not recommend this approach. There is no evidence that this approach is safe or effective, while there is substantial evidence on the safety and effectiveness of benzodiazepines.

Specific Treatment for Severe Symptoms

Treating Delirium Tremens: People with symptoms of delirium tremens must be treated immediately. Untreated delirium tremens has a fatality rate that can be as high as 20%. Treatment usually involves intravenous antianxiety medications. It is extremely important that fluids be administered. Restraints may be necessary to prevent injury to the patient or to others.

Treating Seizures: Seizures are usually self-limited and treated with a benzodiazepine. Intravenous phenytoin (Dilantin) along with a benzodiazepine may be used in patients who have a history of seizures, who have epilepsy, or in those with ongoing seizures. Because phenytoin may lower blood pressure, the patient's heart should be monitored during treatment. Chlormethiazole, a derivative of vitamin B1, is used in Europe for reducing agitation and seizures.

Psychosis: For hallucinations or extremely aggressive behavior, antipsychotic drugs, particularly haloperidol (Haldol), may be administered. Korsakoff's psychosis (Wernicke-Korsakoff syndrome) is caused by severe vitamin B1 (thiamine) deficiencies, which cannot be replaced orally. Rapid and immediate injection of the B vitamin thiamin is necessary.

Therapy

Standard forms of therapy for alcoholism include:

• Cognitive-behavioral therapy;

• Combined behavioral intervention;

• Interactional group psychotherapy based on the Alcoholics Anonymous (AA) 12-step program.

Comparison studies have reported that these approaches are equally effective when the program is competently administered. Specific people may do better with one program than another. One study, for example, examined the differences in success rates on type 1 or type 2 alcoholics:

Categories Of Alcoholic Types   ♣ It's A Fact!!

Some researchers have categorized people with alcoholism as Type 1 or Type 2.

• Type 1 individuals are more often women. They typically become alcoholic at a later age, have less severe symptoms or fewer psychiatric problems, and have a better outlook on life than those classified as type 2.

• Type 2 people are more likely to be male. They tend to become alcoholic at an early age and have a high family risk for alcoholism, more severe symptoms, and a negative outlook on life.

Not only do these two groups tend to respond differently to psychotherapeutic approaches, but they may also respond differently to medications.

Source: © 2007 A.D.A.M., Inc. Reprinted with permission.

- People in the type 1 group did well with the 12-step approach. They did not do as well with cognitive-behavioral therapy. (Type 1 individuals become alcoholic at a later age, have less severe symptoms or fewer psychiatric problems, and have a better outlook on life than those classified as type 2. They are more likely to be women.)

- The people in the type 2 group tended to do better with cognitive-behavioral therapy. (Type 2 people are more likely to be male, become alcoholic at an early age, have a high family risk for alcoholism, have more severe symptoms, and have a negative outlook on life.)

This difference in response to the two forms of treatment held up after two years. Other studies have also reported that people with fewer psychiatric problems do best with the AA approach.

Interactional Group Psychotherapy (Alcoholics Anonymous)

AA, founded in 1935, is an excellent example of interactional group psychotherapy and remains the most well-known program for helping people with alcoholism. It offers a very strong support network using group meetings open seven days a week in locations all over the world. A buddy system, group understanding of alcoholism, and forgiveness for relapses are AA's standard methods for building self-worth and alleviating feelings of isolation.

> ♣ **It's A Fact!!**
>
> Researchers speculate that fewer marital, family, or work responsibilities among younger persons may help explain why persons diagnosable with alcohol dependence at early ages are less likely to recognize and seek treatment for their drinking-related problems. They also note that, because episodes of heavy drinking are more common among youth in general, those with early dependence onset may be less likely to recognize their dependence.
>
> Source: "Early Alcohol Dependence Linked to Reduced Treatment Seeking and Chronic Relapse," NIAAA, September 2006.

AA's 12-step approach to recovery includes a spiritual component that might deter people who lack religious convictions. Prayer and meditation, however, have been known to be of great value in the healing process of many diseases, even in people with no particular religious assignation. AA emphasizes that the "higher power" component of its program need not refer to any specific belief system. Associated membership programs, Al-Anon and Alateen, offer help for family members and friends.

The 12 Steps Of Alcoholics Anonymous

1. We admit we were powerless over alcohol—that our lives have become unmanageable.

2. We have come to believe that a Power greater than ourselves could restore us to sanity.

3. We have made a decision to turn our will and our lives over to the care of God, as we understand what this Power is.

4. We have made a searching and fearless moral inventory of ourselves.

5. We have admitted to God, to ourselves, and to another human being the exact nature of our wrongs.

6. We are entirely ready to have God remove all these defects of character.

7. We have humbly asked God to remove our shortcomings.

8. We have made a list of all persons we had harmed and have become willing to make amends to them all.

9. We have made direct amends to such people wherever possible, except when to do so would injure them or others.

10. We have continued to take personal inventory and when we were wrong promptly admitted it.

11. We have sought through prayer and meditation to improve our conscious contact with God as we understand what this higher Power is, praying only for knowledge of God's will for us and the power to carry that out.

12. Having had a spiritual awakening as the result of these steps, we have tried to carry this message to alcoholics and to practice these principles in all our affairs.

Cognitive-Behavioral Therapy

Cognitive-behavioral therapy (CBT) uses a structured teaching approach and may be better than AA for people with severe alcoholism. Patients are given instruction and homework assignments intended to improve their ability to cope with basic living situations, control their behavior, and change the way they think about drinking. The following are examples of approaches:

• Patients might write a history of their drinking experiences and describe what they consider to be risky situations.

• They are then assigned activities to help them cope when exposed to "cues" (places or circumstances that trigger their desire to drink).

• Patients may also be given tasks that are designed to replace drinking. An interesting and successful example of such a program was one that enlisted patients in a softball team. This gave them the opportunity to practice coping skills, develop supportive relationships, and engage in healthy alternative activities.

CBT may be especially effective when used in combination with opioid antagonists, such as naltrexone. CBT that addresses alcoholism and depression also may be an important treatment for patients with both conditions.

Combined Behavioral Intervention

Combined behavioral intervention (CBI) is a new form of therapy that uses special counseling techniques to help motivate people with alcoholism to change their drinking behavior. CBI combines elements from other psychotherapy treatments such as cognitive behavioral therapy, motivational enhancement therapy, and 12-step programs. Patients are taught how to cope with drinking triggers. Patients also learn strategies for refusing alcohol so that they can achieve and maintain abstinence. In a 2006 study in the *Journal of the American Medical Association*, CBI—combined with regular doctor's office visits (medical management)—worked as well as naltrexone in successfully treating alcoholism.

Behavioral Therapies For Partners

Partners of people with alcoholism can also benefit greatly from behavioral approaches that help them cope with their mate. Children of an alcoholic mother or father may do better if both parents participate in couples-based therapy, rather than just treating the parent with alcoholism.

Treating Sleep Disturbances

Nearly all patients who are alcohol dependent suffer from insomnia and sleep problems, which can last months to years after abstinence. Sleep disturbances may even be important factors in relapse. Available therapies include sleep hygiene, bright light therapy, meditation, relaxation methods, and other nondrug approaches. Many medications for inducing sleep are not recommended in people with alcoholism.

Alternative Methods

Some people try alternative methods, such as acupuncture or hypnosis. Such approaches are not harmful. In one study, acupuncture reduced the desire for alcohol in nearly half of people, although it was not significantly more helpful than conventional treatments.

Medications

In the U.S., three drugs are specifically approved to treat alcohol dependence:

- Naltrexone (ReVia, Vivitrol)
- Acamprosate (Campral)
- Disulfiram (Antabuse)

Naltrexone and acamprosate are categorized as anticraving drugs. Disulfiram is an aversion drug. Other types of medications, such as antidepressants, may also be used to treat patients with alcoholism.

Anticraving Medications

Anticraving drugs are opioid antagonists. These drugs reduce the intoxicating effects of alcohol and the urge to drink

Naltrexone: Naltrexone (ReVia, Vivitrol) is approved for the treatment of alcoholism and helps reduce alcohol dependence in the short term for people with low-to-moderate alcohol dependency. ReVia is a pill that is taken daily by mouth. In 2006, the FDA approved Vivitrol, a once-a-month injectable form of naltrexone.

Naltrexone is usually prescribed along with psychotherapy. The most common side effect is nausea, which is usually mild and temporary. High doses can cause liver damage. The drug should not be given to anyone who has used narcotics within seven to ten days. For ReVia, it is important that patients take the pill on a daily basis. Because many patients have difficulty sticking to this daily regimen, a monthly injection of Vivitrol may be an easier option.

Naltrexone does not work in all patients. Some studies suggest that people with a specific genetic variant may respond better to the drug than those without the gene. The gene regulates receptors that affect the response to opioids. A 2005 study indicated that naltrexone works best for patients who have a family history of alcoholism, began drinking at an early age, and abuse other drugs.

Research is being conducted on the effects of combining naltrexone with acamprosate (Campral), particularly for individuals who have not responded to single drug treatment. In a 2006 study in the *Journal of the American Medical Association* that examined various outpatient drug and behavioral treatments, naltrexone worked as well as psychotherapy in preventing relapse to heavy drinking for patients who had recently abstained from alcohol. However, the study showed no benefit for acamprosate either when combined with naltrexone or used alone.

Acamprosate: Acamprosate (Campral) is the newest drug to be approved for treatment of alcoholism. Acamprosate calms the brain and reduces cravings by inhibiting the transmission of the neurotransmitter gamma aminobutyric acid (GABA). Studies indicate that it reduces the frequency of drinking and, in concert with psychotherapy, improves quality of life even in patients with severe alcohol dependence. One study reported that 60% of patients remained abstinent for 12 weeks, and in another 43% were still abstinent after nearly a year. The drug may cause occasional diarrhea and headache. It also can impair certain memory functions but does not alter short-term working memory or mood. People with kidney problems should use acamprosate cautiously. For some patients, combination therapy with naltrexone or disulfiram may provide greater benefit than acamprosate alone.

Aversion Medications

Disulfiram: Some drugs have properties that interact with alcohol to produce distressing side effects. Disulfiram (Antabuse) causes flushing, headache, nausea, and vomiting if a person drinks alcohol while taking the drug. The symptoms can be triggered after drinking half a glass of wine or half a shot of liquor and may last from half an hour to two hours, depending on dosage of the drug and the amount of alcohol consumed. One dose of disulfiram is usually effective for one to two weeks. Overdose can be dangerous, causing low blood pressure, chest pain, shortness of breath, and even death. The drug is more effective if patients have family or social support, including AA "buddies," who are close by and vigilant to ensure that they take it.

Other Drugs

Topiramate: Topiramate (Topamax) is an anti-seizure drug used to treat epilepsy. It also helps control impulsivity. Studies indicate it may be a promising treatment for alcohol dependence. In one well-designed study, patients who took topiramate had fewer heavy drinking days, fewer drinks per day, and more continuous days of abstinence than patients who received placebo. Side effects included burning and itching skin sensations, change in taste sensation, loss of appetite, and difficulty concentrating.

Chapter 32

Understanding Alcohol Withdrawal And Delirium Tremens

Alcohol Withdrawal

Definition: Alcohol withdrawal refers to symptoms that may occur when a person who has been drinking too much alcohol every day suddenly stops drinking alcohol.

Causes: Alcohol withdrawal usually occurs in adults, but it may happen in teenagers or children as well. It can occur when a person who uses alcohol excessively suddenly stops drinking alcohol. The withdrawal usually occurs within 5–10 hours after the last drink, but it may occur up to 7–10 days later.

Excessive alcohol use is generally considered the equivalent of 2–6 pints of beer (or four ounces of "hard" alcohol) per day for one week, or habitual use of alcohol that disrupts a person's life and routines.

Symptoms: Mild-to-moderate psychological symptoms:

• Jumpiness or nervousness

• Shakiness

About This Chapter: This chapter includes information from "Alcohol Withdrawal," May 18, 2007; and "Delirium Tremens," January 22, 2007; both documents © 2007 A.D.A.M., Inc. Reprinted with permission.

- Anxiety

- Irritability or easy excitability

- Rapid emotional changes

- Depression

- Fatigue

- Difficulty thinking clearly

- Bad dreams

Mild-to-moderate physical symptoms:

- Headache: general, pulsating

- Sweating: especially the palms of the hands or the face

- Nausea and vomiting

- Loss of appetite

- Insomnia (sleeping difficulty)

- Pallor

- Rapid heart rate

- Eye pupils enlarged (dilated pupils)

- Clammy skin

- Tremor of the hands

- Involuntary, abnormal movements of the eyelids

Severe symptoms:

- Delirium tremens: a state of confusion and visual hallucinations

- Agitation

- Fever

- Convulsions

♣ **It's A Fact!!**
The more heavily a person had been drinking every day, the more likely that person will develop alcohol withdrawal symptoms when they stop. The likelihood of developing severe withdrawal symptoms also increases if a person has other medical problems.

Source: © May 18, 2007, A.D.A.M., Inc. Reprinted with permission.

- Black outs: when the person forgets what happened during the drinking episode

Exams and tests: The health care provider will check for:

- Rapid heartbeat (tachycardia)

- Rapid breathing (tachypnea)

- Elevated temperature

- Abnormal eye movements

- Shaky hands

- General body shaking

- Abnormal heart rhythms

- Internal bleeding

- Liver failure

- Dehydration

A toxicology screen may be performed as well as other blood tests.

Treatment: The goals are to treat the immediate withdrawal symptoms, prevent complications, and begin long-term preventative therapy.

- The person will probably have to stay at the hospital for constant observation. Heart rate, breathing, body temperature, and blood pressure are monitored, as well as fluids and electrolytes (chemicals in the body such as sodium and potassium).

- The patient's symptoms may progress rapidly and may quickly become life-threatening. Drugs that depress the central nervous system (such as sedatives) may be required to reduce symptoms, often in moderately large doses.

- Treatment may require maintenance of a moderately sedated state for a week or more until withdrawal is complete. A class of medications known as the benzodiazepines are often useful in reducing a range of symptoms.

- A drying-out period may be appropriate. No alcohol is allowed during this time.

- The health care provider will watch closely for signs of delirium tremens.

- Hallucinations that occur without other symptoms or complications are uncommon. They are treated with hospitalization and antipsychotic medications as needed.

- Testing and treatment for other medical problems associated with use of alcohol is necessary. This may include disorders such as alcoholic liver disease, blood clotting disorders, alcoholic neuropathy, heart disorders (such as alcoholic cardiomyopathy), chronic brain syndromes (such as Wernicke-Korsakoff syndrome), and malnutrition.

♣ **It's A Fact!!**

Outlook (prognosis): Alcohol withdrawal may range from a mild and uncomfortable disorder to a serious, life-threatening condition. Symptoms usually begin within 12 hours of the last drink. The symptoms peak in 48–72 hours and may persist for a week or more.

Symptoms such as sleep changes, rapid changes in mood, and fatigue may last for three to 12 months or more. If a person continues to drink excessively, they may develop many medical conditions such as liver and heart disease.

Source: © May 18, 2007, A.D.A.M., Inc. Reprinted with permission.

Rehabilitation for alcoholism is often recommended. This may include social support such as Alcoholics Anonymous, medications, and behavior therapy.

When To Contact A Medical Professional: Call your health care provider or go the emergency room if symptoms indicate alcohol withdrawal, especially in a person who has a history of habitual use of alcohol, or a history of stopping use of alcohol after a period of heavy alcohol consumption. Alcohol withdrawal is a serious condition that may rapidly become life threatening.

- Call for an appointment with your health care provider if symptoms persist after treatment.

- Go to the emergency room or call the local emergency number (such as 911) if potentially lethal symptoms occur, including seizures, fever, delirium or severe confusion, hallucinations, and irregular heart beat.

Prevention: Minimize or avoid the use of alcohol. In people with alcoholism, total abstinence from alcohol may be necessary.

Delirium Tremens

Definition: Delirium tremens is a severe form of alcohol withdrawal that involves sudden and severe mental or neurological changes.

Alternative Names: DTs; Alcohol withdrawal-delirium tremens

Causes: Delirium tremens can occur after a period of heavy alcohol drinking, especially when the person does not eat enough food. It may also be triggered by head injury, infection, or illness in people with a history of heavy alcohol use.

It is most common in people who have a history of alcohol withdrawal. It is especially common in those who drink the equivalent of seven to eight pints of beer (or one pint of "hard" alcohol) every day for several months. Delirium tremens also commonly affects those who have had a history of habitual alcohol use or alcoholism for more than 10 years.

Symptoms:

- Body tremors
- Mental status changes
    - Agitation, irritability
    - Confusion, disorientation
    - Decreased attention span
    - Decreased mental status, such as deep sleep that persists for a day or longer; stupor, sleepiness, lethargy; usually occurs after acute symptoms

- Delirium (severe, acute loss of mental functions)
- Excitement
- Fear
- Hallucinations (visual hallucinations such as seeing things that are not present are most common)
- Highly sensitive to light, sound, touch (sensory hyperacuity)
- Increased activity
- Mood changes rapidly
- Restlessness, excitement

- Seizures
  - Most common in first 24–48 hours after last alcohol consumption
  - Most common in people with previous complications from alcohol withdrawal
  - Usually generalized tonic-clonic seizures

- Symptoms of alcohol withdrawal
  - Anxiety
  - Depression
  - Difficulty thinking clearly
  - Fatigue
  - Feeling jumpy or nervous
  - Feeling shaky
  - Headache, general, pulsating
  - Insomnia (difficulty falling and staying asleep)
  - Irritability or easily excited
  - Loss of appetite
  - Nausea
  - Pale skin
  - Palpitations (sensation of feeling the heart beat)

- Rapid emotional changes
- Sweating, especially the palms of the hands or the face
- Vomiting

Additional symptoms that may occur:

- Chest pain
- Fever
- Stomach pain

Symptoms most commonly occur within 72 hours after the last drink. However, they may occur up to seven to 10 days after the last drink. Symptoms may get worse rapidly.

Exams And Tests: Delirium tremens is a medical emergency. The health care provider will perform a physical exam. Signs may include:

- Heavy sweating
- Increased startle reflex
- Irregular heartbeat
- Problems with eye muscle movement
- Rapid heart rate
- Rapid muscle tremors

The following tests may be done:

- Chem-20
- Electrocardiogram (ECG)
- Electroencephalogram (EEG)
- Toxicology screen

Treatment: The goals of treatment are to:

- Save the person's life
- Relieve symptoms
- Prevent complications

A hospital stay is required. The health care team will regularly check:

- Blood chemistry results, such as electrolyte levels
- Fluids
- Vital signs (temperature, pulse, rate of breathing, blood pressure)

Symptoms such as seizures and heart arrhythmias are treated with the following medications:

- Anticonvulsants such as phenytoin or phenobarbital
- Central nervous system depressants such as diazepam
- Clonidine to reduce cardiovascular symptoms and reduce anxiety
- Sedatives

The patient may need to be put into a sedated state for a week or more until withdrawal is complete. Benzodiazepine medications such as diazepam or lorazepam are often used. These drugs also help treat seizures, anxiety, and tremors. Antipsychotic medications such as haloperidol may sometimes be necessary for persons with hallucinations.

Long-term preventive treatment may begin after the patient recovers from acute symptoms. This may involve a "drying out" period, in which no alcohol is allowed. The person should receive treatment for alcohol use or alcoholism, including:

- Counseling
- Support groups (such as Alcoholics Anonymous)

The patient should be tested, and if necessary, treated for other medical problems associated with alcohol use. Such problems may include:

- Alcoholic cardiomyopathy
- Alcoholic liver disease
- Alcoholic neuropathy
- Blood clotting disorders
- Wernicke-Korsakoff syndrome

Possible complications:

• Heart arrhythmias, may be life threatening

• Injury from falls during seizures

• Injury to self or others caused by mental state (confusion/delirium)

• Seizures

When To Contact A Medical Professional: Go to the emergency room or call the local emergency number (such as 911) if you have symptoms. Delirium tremens is an emergency condition.

Prevention: Avoid or reduce the use of alcohol. Get prompt medical treatment for symptoms of alcohol withdrawal.

♣ It's A Fact!!

Outlook (prognosis): Delirium tremens is serious and may be life threatening. Symptoms such as sleeplessness, feeling tired, and emotional instability may persist for a year or more.

Source: © January 22, 2007, A.D.A.M., Inc. Reprinted with permission.

Chapter 33

Dealing With Addiction

Jason's life is beginning to unravel. His grades have slipped, he's moody, he doesn't talk to his friends, and he has stopped showing up for practice. Jason's friends know he has been experimenting with drugs and now they're worried he has become addicted.

Defining an addiction is tricky, and knowing how to handle one is even harder.

What Are Substance Abuse And Addiction?

The difference between substance abuse and addiction is very slight. Substance abuse means using an illegal substance or using a legal substance in the wrong way. Addiction begins as abuse, or using a substance like marijuana or cocaine. You can abuse a drug (or alcohol) without having an addiction. For example, just because Sara smoked weed a few times doesn't mean that she has an addiction, but it does mean that she's abusing a drug—and that could lead to an addiction.

People can get addicted to all sorts of substances. When we think of addiction, we usually think of alcohol or illegal drugs. But people become addicted to medications, cigarettes, even glue! And some substances are more addictive than others: Drugs like crack or heroin are so addictive that they might only be used once or twice before the user loses control.

Addiction means a person has no control over whether he or she uses a drug or drinks. Someone who's addicted to cocaine has grown so used to the drug that he or she has to have it. Addiction can be physical, psychological, or both.

Physical addiction is when a person's body actually becomes dependent on a particular substance (even smoking is physically addictive). It also means building tolerance to that substance, so that a person needs a larger dose than ever before to get the same effects. Someone who is physically addicted and stops using a substance like drugs, alcohol, or cigarettes may experience withdrawal symptoms. Common symptoms of withdrawal are diarrhea, shaking, and generally feeling awful.

❖ It's A Fact!!
Researchers are finding common genetic factors in alcohol and nicotine addiction, which may explain, in part, why alcoholics are often smokers. Alcoholics who smoke compound their health problems. More alcoholics die from tobacco-related illnesses, such as heart disease or cancer, than from chronic liver disease, cirrhosis, or other conditions that are more directly tied to excessive drinking. Abuse of other substances is also common among alcoholics.

Source: Excerpted from "Alcoholism," © 2007 A.D.A.M., Inc. Reprinted with permission.

Psychological addiction happens when the cravings for a drug are psychological or emotional. People who are psychologically addicted feel overcome by the desire to have a drug. They may lie or steal to get it.

A person crosses the line between abuse and addiction when he or she is no longer trying the drug to have fun or get high, but has come to depend on it. His or her whole life centers around the need for the drug. An addicted person—whether it's a physical or psychological addiction or both—no longer feels like there is a choice in taking a substance.

Signs Of Addiction

The most obvious sign of an addiction is the need to have a particular drug or substance. However, many other signs can suggest a possible addiction, such as changes in mood or weight loss or gain. (These also are signs of other conditions, too, though, such as depression or eating disorders.)

Signs that you or someone you know may have a drug or alcohol addiction include:

Psychological Signals

- Use of drugs or alcohol as a way to forget problems or to relax
- Withdrawal or keeping secrets from family and friends
- Loss of interest in activities that used to be important
- Problems with schoolwork, such as slipping grades or absences
- Changes in friendships, such as hanging out only with friends who use drugs
- Spending a lot of time figuring out how to get drugs
- Stealing or selling belongings to be able to afford drugs
- Failed attempts to stop taking drugs or drinking
- Anxiety, anger, or depression
- Mood swings

Physical Signals

- Changes in sleeping habits
- Feeling shaky or sick when trying to stop
- Needing to take more of the substance to get the same effect
- Changes in eating habits, including weight loss or gain

Getting Help

If you think you're addicted to drugs or alcohol, recognizing that you have a problem is the first step in getting help.

A lot of people think they can kick the problem on their own, but that doesn't work for most people. Find someone you trust to talk to. It may help to talk to a friend or someone your own age at first, but a supportive and understanding adult is your best option for getting help. If you can't talk to your parents, you might want to approach a school counselor, relative, doctor, favorite teacher, or religious leader.

♣ It's A Fact!!
What Causes Relapse?

Social And Emotional Causes Of Alcoholic Relapse: Between 80–90% of people treated for alcoholism relapse, even after years of abstinence. Patients and their caregivers should understand that relapses of alcoholism are analogous to recurrent flare-ups of chronic physical diseases. Factors that place a person at high risk for relapse include:

- Frustration and anger

- Social pressure

- Internal temptation

Mental And Emotional Stress: Alcohol blocks out emotional pain and is often perceived as a loyal friend when human relationships fail. It is also associated with freedom and with a loss of inhibition that offsets the tedium of daily routines. When the alcoholic tries to quit drinking, the brain seeks to restore what it perceives to be its equilibrium. The brain's best weapons to achieve this are depression, anxiety, and stress (the emotional equivalents of physical pain), which are produced by brain chemical imbalances. These negative moods continue to tempt alcoholics to return to drinking long after physical withdrawal symptoms have abated.

It is important to realize that any life change, even changes for the better, may cause temporary grief and anxiety. With time and the substitution of healthier pleasures, this emotional turmoil weakens and can be overcome.

Co-Dependency: Many aspects of the ex-drinker's relationships change when drinking stops, making it difficult to remain abstinent:

Unfortunately, overcoming addiction is not easy. Quitting drugs or drinking is probably going to be one of the hardest things you've ever done. It's not a sign of weakness if you need professional help from a trained drug counselor or therapist. Most people who try to kick a drug or alcohol problem need professional assistance or a treatment program to do so.

- One of the most difficult problems that occur is being around other people who are able to drink socially without danger of addiction. A sense of isolation, a loss of enjoyment, and the ex-drinker's belief that pity, not respect, is guiding a friend's attitude can lead to loneliness, low self-esteem, and a strong desire to drink again.

- Friends may not easily accept the sober, perhaps more subdued, ex-drinker. Close friends and even intimate partners may have difficulty in changing their responses to this newly sober person and, even worse, may encourage a return to drinking.

- To preserve marriages, spouses of alcoholics often build their own self-images on surviving or handling their mates' difficult behavior and then discover that they find it difficult to adjust to new roles and behaviors. In such cases, separation from these "enablers" may be necessary for survival. It is no wonder that, when faced with such losses, even if they are temporary, a person returns to drinking. The best course in these cases is to encourage close friends and family members to seek help as well. Fortunately, groups such as Al-Anon exist for this purpose.

Social And Cultural Pressures: The media portrays the pleasures of drinking in advertising and programming. The medical benefits of light-to-moderate drinking are frequently publicized, giving ex-drinkers the spurious excuse of returning to alcohol for their health. These messages must be categorically ignored and acknowledged for what they are: An industry's attempt to profit from potentially great harm to individuals.

Source: Excerpted from "Alcoholism," © 2007 A.D.A.M., Inc. Reprinted with permission.

Once you start a treatment program, try these tips to make the road to recovery less bumpy:

- Tell your friends about your decision to stop using drugs. Your true friends will respect your decision. This might mean that you need to find a new group of friends who will be 100% supportive. Unless everyone decides to kick their drug habit at once, you probably won't be able to hang out with the friends you did drugs with before.

- Ask your friends or family to be available when you need them. You may need to call someone in the middle of the night just to talk. If you're going through a tough time, don't try to handle things on your own—accept the help your family and friends offer.

- Accept invitations only to events that you know won't involve drugs or alcohol. Going to the movies is probably safe, but you may want to skip a Friday night party until you're feeling more secure. Plan activities that don't involve drugs. Go to the movies, try bowling, or take an art class with a friend.

- Have a plan about what you'll do if you find yourself in a place with drugs or alcohol. The temptation will be there sometimes, but if you know how you're going to handle it, you'll be OK. Establish a plan with your parents or siblings so that if you call home using a code, they'll know that your call is a signal you need a ride out of there.

- Remind yourself that having an addiction doesn't make you bad or weak. If you fall back into old patterns (backslide) a bit, talk to an adult as soon as possible. There's nothing to be ashamed about, but it's important to get help soon so that all of the hard work you put into your recovery is not lost.

If you're worried about a friend who has an addiction, use these tips to help him or her, too. For example, let your friend know that you are available to talk or offer your support. If you notice a friend backsliding, talk about it openly and ask what you can do to help. If your friend is going back to drugs or drinking and won't accept your help, don't be afraid to talk to a nonthreatening, understanding adult, like your parent or school counselor. It may seem like you're ratting your friend out, but it's the best support you can offer.

Above all, offer a friend who's battling an addiction lots of encouragement and praise. It may seem corny, but hearing that you care is just the kind of motivation your friend needs.

Staying Clean

Recovering from a drug or alcohol addiction doesn't end with a 6-week treatment program. It's a lifelong process. Many people find that joining a support group can help them stay clean. There are support groups specifically for teens and younger people. You'll meet people who have gone through the same experiences you have, and you'll be able to participate in real-life discussions about drugs that you won't hear in your school's health class.

Many people find that helping others is also the best way to help themselves. Your understanding of how difficult the recovery process can be will help you to support others—both teens and adults—who are battling an addiction.

☞ Remember!!

If you do have a relapse, recognizing the problem as soon as possible is critical. Get help right away so that you don't undo all the hard work you put into your initial recovery. And, if you do have a relapse, don't ever be afraid to ask for help!

Source: © 2007 Nemours Foundation.

Part Five

Preventing Teen Alcohol Use

Chapter 34

Adolescent Drinking: Prevention And Intervention Programs

Young Adult Drinking

Young adulthood is a time when many people establish lifelong patterns of alcohol use (or nonuse). Others take a different course, maybe drinking heavily in their late teens or young adult years, then maturing out of risky alcohol use as they begin to assume more adult roles. By identifying common tracks or trajectories of alcohol use and abuse across adolescence and young adulthood, researchers are hoping to better understand how problems with alcohol begin and how they are likely to develop over time in order to plan effective prevention and intervention programs.

So far, studies of alcohol use trajectories have yielded several important findings. For example, although the majority of young adults report drinking some alcohol, anywhere from one-third to two-thirds report that they

About This Chapter: This chapter begins with excerpts from "Alcohol Alert: Young Adult Drinking," National Institute on Alcohol Abuse and Alcoholism (NIAAA), April 2006. Additional text under the heading "Selected Prevention Intervention Programs" was excerpted from the descriptions of currently reviewed programs (2006–2008) designed to address the concerns of underage and binge drinking. Further information about these programs can be found through the Substance Abuse and Mental Health Services Administration (SAMHSA)'s National Registry of Evidence-Based Programs and Practices, available online at http://nrepp.samhsa.gov.

never drink heavily. And most people tend to reduce their drinking by their mid-twenties as they start to acquire adult roles, such as becoming a spouse, parent, and worker.

Prevention And Intervention

What researchers have learned about the different trajectories that drinkers follow as they progress through young adulthood has important implications for prevention. Studies have shown that (1) people follow a variety of pathways across the adolescent and young adult years, (2) alcohol use behaviors change differently for different people, and (3) factors that predict alcohol use patterns emerge and disappear at different ages. One approach to prevention simply will not fit every need. Recognizing the varied and ever-changing trajectories that alcohol use can take offers scientists a solid developmental foundation on which to build effective interventions.

♣ It's A Fact!!

The age when people begin drinking (especially heavy drinking) has proven to be an especially good predictor of problems with alcohol later in life. Interviews of adults consistently confirm a strong association between an early initiation of drinking and later alcohol-related problems. People who binge drink also are at higher risk for later alcohol problems, and young adults who drink heavily are at particular risk for behavioral problems and may have trouble adjusting to adult roles.

One way to prevent alcohol-related problems—among young people or the population as a whole—is to establish policies that reduce overall alcohol consumption rates or reduce the rates of high-risk drinking. Alcohol control policies influence the availability of alcohol, the social messages about drinking that are conveyed by advertising and other marketing approaches, and the enforcement of existing alcohol laws.

Most alcohol control policies target either young people under the legal drinking age of 21 or the drinking behavior of the population as a whole, rather than specific subpopulations such as young adults. Nevertheless, some of these policies have a larger effect on young adult drinkers compared with the rest of the population—for example, measures that address drinking in bars and clubs, because young adults are more likely than other age groups to patronize these establishments.

Prevention On College Campuses: In recent years, an increasing number of colleges have implemented policies to reduce alcohol consumption and alcohol-related problems. Examples include establishing alcohol-free college residences and campuses, prohibiting self-service of alcohol at campus events, prohibiting beer kegs on campus, and banning sales or marketing of alcohol on campus. Though research on the success of these programs is limited, studies have shown that students living in substance-free residences are less likely to engage in heavy episodic or binge drinking (five or more drinks in one sitting for men, four or more for women), and underage students at colleges that ban alcohol are less likely to engage in heavy episodic drinking and more likely to abstain from alcohol. College alcohol policies are less likely to have an effect on students who live off campus than on, however.

Prevention In The Military: Current strategies to prevent alcohol problems among military personnel are similar to strategies being used with other populations of drinkers, including instituting and enforcing policies that regulate alcohol availability and pricing, deglamorizing alcohol use, and promoting personal responsibility and overall good health.

Prevention Among The General Population: Some of the principal strategies for influencing the drinking behavior of the general population are raising taxes on alcoholic beverages, limiting the number of alcohol establishments in a particular geographic area, training the staff of bars and stores to sell alcohol responsibly, and restricting alcohol marketing and advertising.

Of these strategies, the effects of raising alcohol prices have been the most extensively studied. The most common method of raising prices is to increase federal, state, or local taxes on alcoholic beverages. Studies show that underage youth are particularly sensitive to increased prices, decreasing their alcohol consumption by a greater amount than older drinkers. A few studies have looked at how alcohol prices affect drinking among college students and young adults. One study showed that college students faced with higher alcohol prices were less likely to transition from being abstainers to moderate drinkers and from moderate to heavy drinkers. Another study found that low sale prices were associated with higher rates of heavy episodic drinking among college students.

Prevention Of Drinking And Driving: Traffic crashes are the leading cause of death among teens, and more than half of drivers ages 21–24 who died in traffic crashes in 2003 tested positive for alcohol. Raising the minimum legal drinking age (MLDA) to 21 has produced significant reductions in traffic crashes among 18- to 20-year-olds, and it appears to have had a spillover effect on the drinking behavior of 21- to 25-year-olds. One study found that college students who had been high school seniors in states when the MLDA was 18 drank more while in college than their counterparts who had been high school seniors in states with an MLDA of 21. High school graduates of the same age who were not attending college also drank more on average if they had been seniors in states with an MLDA of 18.

Another effective strategy to reduce drinking and driving is to lower the legal limit for allowable blood alcohol content (BAC) for drivers. In the past two decades, all states in the United States have adopted a BAC limit of 0.08 percent for adult drivers and a BAC limit of zero, or slightly higher*, for youth under age 21. These often are referred to as "zero tolerance" laws. (*Most laws use a 0.02-percent limit rather than an absolute zero limit to allow for small measurement errors in BAC test instruments and to avoid challenges from youth who claim they have taken medication with small amounts of alcohol).

- Studies have found that laws setting the legal allowable BAC at 0.08 percent have resulted in five-percent to eight-percent reductions in alcohol-related fatal traffic crashes among all drivers.

- Laws setting the limit at 0.02 percent have led to a 19-percent reduction in drinking and driving and a 20-percent reduction in fatal traffic crashes among young drivers.

Comprehensive Community Prevention Approaches: Perhaps the best way to reduce harmful drinking and alcohol-related problems in young adults is through comprehensive approaches that rely heavily on community action. Whether they are working, attending college, or in the military, young adults typically are part of a community. And young people's usual sources of alcohol—retail outlets, restaurants, bars, and social settings such as parties—also operate within the environment of the community.

To be effective, community prevention interventions require a mix of research-tested programs and policy strategies, along with strong enforcement of those laws. Three National Institute on Alcohol Abuse and Alcoholism (NIAAA)-sponsored community trial projects have been extensively studied and are showing promise: The Saving Lives Project, the Community Trials Project, and Communities Mobilizing for Change on Alcohol. These trials provide strong evidence for the positive effects of research-based local prevention efforts that take a comprehensive approach using a variety of strategies.

Selected Prevention And Intervention Programs

Across Ages
Date of Review: June 2008
http://nrepp.samhsa.gov/programfulldetails.asp?PROGRAM_ID=148

Across Ages is a school- and community-based substance abuse prevention program for youth ages 9 to 13. The unique feature of Across Ages is the pairing of older adult mentors (55 years and older) with young adolescents, specifically those making the transition to middle school. The overall goal of the program is to increase protective factors for high-risk students to prevent, reduce, or delay the use of alcohol, tobacco, and other drugs and the problems associated with substance use.

All Stars
Date of Review: June 2007
http://nrepp.samhsa.gov/programfulldetails.asp?PROGRAM_ID=129

All Stars is a multiyear school-based program for middle school students (11 to 14 years old) designed to prevent and delay the onset of high-risk behaviors such as drug use, violence, and premature sexual activity. The program focuses on five topics important to preventing high-risk behaviors: (1) developing positive ideals that do not fit with high-risk behavior; (2) creating a belief in conventional norms; (3) building strong personal commitments; (4) bonding with school, prosocial institutions, and family; and (5) increasing positive parental attentiveness.

CASASTART

Date of Review: May 2007
http://nrepp.samhsa.gov/programfulldetails.asp?PROGRAM_ID=121

CASASTART (Striving Together to Achieve Rewarding Tomorrows, formerly known as Children at Risk), is a community-based, school-centered substance abuse and violence prevention program developed by the National Center on Addiction and Substance Abuse at Columbia University (CASA).

CASASTART targets youths between 8 and 13 years old who have a minimum of four identified risk factors. Youth participants may remain in the program up to two years. Specific program objectives of CASASTART include reducing drug and alcohol use, reducing involvement in drug trafficking, decreasing associations with delinquent peers, improving school performance, and reducing violent offenses.

Class Action

Date of Review: April 2007
http://nrepp.samhsa.gov/programfulldetails.asp?PROGRAM_ID=115

Class Action is the second phase of the Project Northland (see below) alcohol-use prevention curriculum series. Class Action (for grades 11–12) and Project Northland (for grades 6–8) are designed to delay the onset of alcohol use, reduce use among youths who have already tried alcohol, and limit the number of alcohol-related problems experienced by young drinkers. Class Action draws upon the social influence theory of behavior change, using interactive, peer-led sessions to explore the real-world legal and social consequences of substance abuse.

Community Trials Intervention To Reduce High-Risk Drinking
Date of Review: February 2008
http://nrepp.samhsa.gov/programfulldetails.asp?PROGRAM_ID=161

Community Trials Intervention To Reduce High-Risk Drinking is a multicomponent, community-based program developed to alter the alcohol use patterns and related problems of people of all ages. The program incorporates a set of environmental interventions that assist communities in (1) using zoning and municipal regulations to restrict alcohol access through alcohol outlet density control; (2) enhancing responsible beverage service by training, testing, and assisting beverage servers and retailers in the development of policies and procedures to reduce intoxication and driving after drinking; (3) increasing law enforcement and sobriety checkpoints to raise actual and perceived risk of arrest for driving after drinking; (4) reducing youth access to alcohol by training alcohol retailers to avoid selling to minors and those who provide alcohol to minors; and (5) forming the coalitions needed to implement and support the interventions that address each of these prevention components. The program aims to help communities reduce alcohol-related accidents and incidents of violence and the injuries that result from them. The program typically is implemented over several years, gradually phasing in various environmental strategies; however, the period of implementation may vary depending on local conditions and goals.

Creating Lasting Family Connections (CLFC)/Creating Lasting Connections (CLC)
Date of Review: June 2007
http://nrepp.samhsa.gov/programfulldetails.asp?PROGRAM_ID=126

Creating Lasting Family Connections (CLFC), the currently available version of Creating Lasting Connections (CLC), is a family-focused program that aims to build the resiliency of youth aged 9 to 17 years and reduce the frequency of their alcohol and other drug (AOD) use. CLFC is designed to be implemented through a community system, such as churches, schools, recreation centers, and court-referred settings. The six modules of the CLFC curriculum, administered to parents/guardians and youth in 18–20 weekly training sessions, focus on imparting knowledge and understanding about the use of alcohol and other drugs, including tobacco; improving communication and conflict resolution skills; building coping mechanisms to resist negative social influences; encouraging the use of community services when personal or family problems arise; engendering self-knowledge, personal responsibility, and respect for others; and delaying the onset and reducing the frequency of AOD use among participating youth. The program emphasizes early intervention services for parents and youth and follow-up case management services for families.

Family Matters
Date of Review: October 2006
http://nrepp.samhsa.gov/programfulldetails.asp?PROGRAM_ID=89

Family Matters is a family-directed program to prevent adolescents 12–14 years of age from using tobacco and alcohol. The intervention is designed to influence population-level prevalence and can be implemented with large numbers of geographically dispersed families. The program encourages communication among family members and focuses on general family characteristics (for example, supervision and communication skills) and substance-specific characteristics (for example, family rules for tobacco and alcohol use and media/peer influences).

Guiding Good Choices
Date of Review: April 2007
http://nrepp.samhsa.gov/programfulldetails.asp?PROGRAM_ID=123

Guiding Good Choices (GGC) is a drug use prevention program that provides parents of children in grades 4 through 8 (9 to 14 years old) with the knowledge and skills needed to guide their children through early adolescence. It seeks to strengthen and clarify family expectations for behavior, enhance the conditions that promote bonding within the family, and teach skills that allow children to resist drug use successfully. GGC is based on research that shows that consistent, positive parental involvement is important to helping children resist substance use and other antisocial behaviors. Formerly known as Preparing for the Drug Free Years, this program was revised in 2003 with more family activities and exercises.

Keepin' It REAL

Date of Review: December 2006

http://nrepp.samhsa.gov/programfulldetails.asp?PROGRAM_ID=119

Keepin' it REAL is a multicultural, school-based substance use prevention program for students 12–14 years old. Keepin' it REAL uses a 10-lesson curriculum taught by trained classroom teachers in 45-minute sessions over 10 weeks, with booster sessions delivered in the following school year.

The curriculum is designed to help students assess the risks associated with substance abuse, enhance decision-making and resistance strategies, improve antidrug normative beliefs and attitudes, and reduce substance use. The narrative and performance-based curriculum draws from communication competence theory and a culturally grounded resiliency model to incorporate traditional ethnic values and practices that protect against substance use. The curriculum places special emphasis on resistance strategies represented in the acronym "REAL" (Refuse offers to use substances, Explain why you do not want to use substances, Avoid situations in which substances are used, and Leave situations in which substances are used).

Lions Quest Skills For Adolescence

Date of Review: January 2007

http://nrepp.samhsa.gov/programfulldetails.asp?PROGRAM_ID=99

Lions Quest Skills for Adolescence (SFA) is a multicomponent, comprehensive life skills education program designed for schoolwide and classroom implementation in grades 6 through 8 (ages 10–14).

The goal of Lions Quest programs is to help young people develop positive commitments to their families, schools, peers, and communities and to encourage healthy, drug-free lives. Lions Quest SFA unites educators, parents, and community members to utilize social influence and social cognitive approaches in developing the following skills and competencies in young adolescents: (1) essential social/emotional competencies, (2) good citizenship skills, (3) strong positive character, (4) skills and attitudes consistent with a drug-free lifestyle and (5) an ethic of service to others within a caring and consistent environment.

Project ALERT

Date of Review: December 2006

http://nrepp.samhsa.gov/programfulldetails.asp?PROGRAM_ID=109

Project ALERT is a school-based prevention program for middle or junior high school students that focuses on alcohol, tobacco, and marijuana use. It seeks to prevent adolescent nonusers from experimenting with these drugs, and to prevent youths who are already experimenting from becoming more regular users or abusers. Based on the social influence model of prevention, the program is designed to help motivate young people to avoid using drugs and to teach them the skills they need to understand and resist prodrug social influences.

Project Northland

Date of Review: March 2007

http://nrepp.samhsa.gov/programfulldetails.asp?PROGRAM_ID=100

Project Northland is a multilevel intervention involving students, peers, parents, and community in programs designed to delay the age at which adolescents begin drinking, reduce alcohol use among those already drinking, and limit the number of alcohol-related problems among young drinkers. Administered to adolescents in grades six through eight on a weekly basis, the program has a specific theme within each grade level that is incorporated into the parent, peer, and community components.

The 6th-grade home-based program targets communication about adolescent alcohol use utilizing student-parent homework assignments, in-class group discussions, and a communitywide task force. The 7th-grade peer- and teacher-led curriculum focuses on resistance skills and normative expectations regarding teen alcohol use, and is implemented through discussions, games, problem-solving tasks, and role-plays. During the first half of the 8th-grade Powerlines peer-led program, students learn about community dynamics related to alcohol use prevention through small group and classroom interactive activities. During the second half, they work on community-based projects and hold a mock town meeting to make community policy recommendations to prevent teen alcohol use.

Project SUCCESS

Date of Review: November 2007

http://nrepp.samhsa.gov/programfulldetails.asp?PROGRAM_ID=199

Project SUCCESS (Schools Using Coordinated Community Efforts to Strengthen Students) is designed to prevent and reduce substance use among students 12 to 18 years of age. The program was originally developed for students attending alternative high schools who are at high risk for substance use and abuse due to poor academic performance, truancy, discipline problems, negative attitudes toward school, and parental substance abuse. In recent years, Project SUCCESS has been used in regular middle and high schools for a broader range of high-risk students.

Project Towards No Drug Abuse

Date of Review: September 2006

http://nrepp.samhsa.gov/programfulldetails.asp?PROGRAM_ID=62

Project Towards No Drug Abuse (Project TND) is a drug use prevention program for high school youth. The current version of the curriculum is designed to help students develop self-control and communication skills, acquire resources that help them resist drug use, improve decision-making strategies, and develop the motivation to not use drugs.

Project Venture

Date of Review: October 2007

http://nrepp.samhsa.gov/programfulldetails.asp?PROGRAM_ID=146

Project Venture is an outdoor experiential youth development program designed primarily for 5th- to 8th-grade American Indian youth. It aims to develop the social and emotional competence that facilitates youths' resistance to alcohol, tobacco, and other drug use. Based on traditional American Indian values such as family, learning from the natural world, spiritual awareness, service to others, and respect, Project Venture's approach is positive and strengths based. The program is designed to foster the development of positive self-concept, effective social interaction skills, a community service ethic, an internal locus of control, and improved decision-making and problem-solving skills.

Protecting You/Protecting Me

Date of Review: March 2008

http://nrepp.samhsa.gov/programfulldetails.asp?PROGRAM_ID=201

Protecting You/Protecting Me (PY/PM) is a 5-year classroom-based alcohol use prevention and vehicle safety program for elementary school students in grades one through five (ages 6–11) and high school students in grades 11 and 12. The program aims to reduce alcohol-related injuries and death among children and youth due to underage alcohol use and riding in vehicles with drivers who are not alcohol free. PY/PM consists of a series of 40 science- and health-based lessons, with eight lessons per year for grades one through five. All lessons are correlated with educational achievement objectives. PY/PM lessons and activities focus on teaching children about (1) the brain—how it continues to develop throughout childhood and adolescence, what alcohol does to the developing brain, and why it is important for children to protect their brains; (2) vehicle safety, particularly what children can do to protect themselves if they have to ride with someone who is not alcohol free; and (3) life skills, including decision-making, stress management, media awareness, resistance strategies, and communication.

STARS For Families

Date of Review: March 2008

http://nrepp.samhsa.gov/programfulldetails.asp?PROGRAM_ID=208

Start Taking Alcohol Risks Seriously (STARS) for Families is a health promotion program that aims to prevent or reduce alcohol use among middle school youth ages 11 to 14 years. The program is founded on the Multi-Component Motivational Stages (McMOS) prevention model, which is based on the stages of behavioral change found within the Transtheoretical Model of Change. The McMOS model posits a continuum of five stages in the initiation of alcohol use: precontemplation (has not tried alcohol in the past year), contemplation (is thinking about trying alcohol soon), preparation (is planning to start drinking soon), action (started drinking in the past six months), and maintenance (has been drinking for longer than six months). STARS for Families intervention materials are tailored to the individual's stage of alcohol use initiation.

STARS for Families has three components. Youth who participate in the program receive brief individual consultations in school or in after-school programs about why and how to avoid alcohol use, and they may also receive a follow-up consultation. These standardized sessions are provided by trained adults guided by protocols. A series of eight postcards are mailed to parents/guardians providing key facts about how to talk to their children about avoiding alcohol. In addition, the family completes four take-home lessons designed to enhance parent-child communication regarding prevention skills and knowledge.

Too Good For Drugs

Date of Review: January 2008
http://nrepp.samhsa.gov/programfulldetails.asp?PROGRAM_ID=215

Too Good for Drugs (TGFD) is a school-based prevention program for kindergarten through 12th grade that builds on students' resiliency by teaching them how to be socially competent and autonomous problem solvers. The program is designed to benefit everyone in the school by providing needed education in social and emotional competencies and by reducing risk factors and building protective factors that affect students in these age groups. TGFD focuses on developing personal and interpersonal skills to resist peer pressures, goal setting, decision-making, bonding with others, having respect for self and others, managing emotions, effective communication, and social interactions. The program also provides information about the negative consequences of drug use and the benefits of a nonviolent, drug-free lifestyle.

Chapter 35

Say No To Alcohol: Handling Peer Pressure

Alcohol: Peer Pressure

If a friend or classmate has ever pushed you into doing something you don't want to do, then you've experienced peer pressure. This is how many young people experiment with underage drinking. If a popular kid offers you a drink, you might think that you'll become popular if you do what he or she says. When a close friend starts drinking, you may worry that you'll lose the friendship if you don't join in.

You may also feel "silent peer pressure" to try drinking. That's when nobody is actually offering you alcohol or encouraging you to try it, but you see other people drinking and feel tempted. This kind of pressure is just as real, but harder to recognize.

There are many ways to handle peer pressure. First, remember these things:

- You don't have to do anything that you don't want to do.

- Giving in to peer pressure is probably not going to magically solve your problems or make people like you.

About This Chapter: This chapter includes information from "Alcohol: Peer Pressure," reprinted with permission from http://pbskids.org/itsmylife, © 2005. All rights reserved. Additional text under the heading "Not Everyone Drinks," is excerpted from "Straight Talk About Alcohol," U.S. Department of Health and Human Services, Office of Women's Health, March 2008.

• It's perfectly okay to say no. You don't owe anyone an explanation.

But let's face it: saying "no" isn't always easy. Most of us worry about fitting in and what others will think of us. If you're worried that you'll lose your friend over a peer pressure situation, you may want to take a closer look at the friendship. A true friend will respect your decisions, and someone who ditches you for not taking orders from them was never a friend to begin with. Also, you may discover that some of your other friends secretly feel the same way you do!

✔ **Quick Tip**

Resisting Spoken Pressure

Spoken pressure—when someone pressures you with words—can be difficult to resist. Most people don't want to risk making others feel bad, but it's important to stand up for yourself. Check out Table 35.1 for strategies to use when dealing with spoken pressure.

Table 35.1. Strategies For Dealing With Spoken Pressure

Do	Don't
Say no assertively	Attend a party unprepared to resist alcohol
Stay alcohol free	Be afraid to say no
Stand up for others	Mumble
Walk away from the situation	Say no too aggressively
Find something else to do with other friends	Act like a know-it-all when saying no

Say no—and let them know you mean it.

- Stand up straight
- Make eye contact
- Say how you feel
- Don't make excuses
- Stick up for yourself

Source: From "The Right To Resist," National Institute on Alcohol Abuse and Alcoholism (NIAAA), April 2006.

If a friend or classmate tries to pressure you, keep in mind why he or she might be doing it:

- He may be trying to make you feel small, so that he can feel better about himself. You don't need his approval to feel good about yourself.

- She may be afraid of anyone who is different from her. You can listen to what she has to say, but that doesn't mean you have to agree with her.

- He could be afraid of criticism, so he'll do the criticizing first. It's better to be alone than to be with someone who is rude to you all the time.

- Deep down, she may be insecure.

- He could be making up rules so that he fits and you don't. Know that there are people who will appreciate you for who you are. Seek them out.

If a simple "No, thanks" won't do the trick, here are some other tactics for turning down someone who is pressuring you to try drinking:

- "I don't like the taste."

- "The smell of alcohol makes me sick and I don't want to smell like that."

- "My parents will ground me if I come home smelling like alcohol."

- "I know someone who died from drinking and I don't want to do it."

- "I don't want to start because I'm trying to get my parents to quit."

- "No thanks, it's not for me."

Whatever you choose, do what feels right for you. Remember: most young people don't drink, so you're in good company! If someone won't stop pressuring you, it's okay to call for backup. Talk to an adult you trust, like your teacher, guidance counselor, your parents, or an older brother or sister.

Not Everyone Drinks

It may seem that everyone around you drinks, especially with alcohol ads all over the place, but there are many teens that do not drink. You do not

✔ **Quick Tip**
Resisting Unspoken Pressure

Sometimes you can feel pressure just from watching how others act or dress, without them saying a word to you. This "unspoken pressure" is especially hard to resist, because instead of standing up to a friend, you're standing up to how you feel inside.

Unspoken pressure may come from role models like your parents, your older siblings, teachers, coaches, or celebrities you see in movies and on TV. Unspoken pressure may also come from peers—your friends or other people your age.

Here are some tips for resisting unspoken pressure.

- Take a reality check—most teens don't drink.
- Remember it's risky—alcohol can be dangerous.
- Walk away from the situation.
- Find something else to do with other friends.

Source: From "The Right To Resist," National Institute on Alcohol Abuse and Alcoholism (NIAAA), April 2006.

need to drink to have fun, be popular, or be comfortable with other people. You can choose to say no to alcohol when friends want to drink. Here are some ways to say no.

- Just say, "No thanks" or "I don't drink."
- Don't go to places where there will be drinking. Suggest another activity to do. You can catch a movie, go out to dinner, go shopping, go see a school play, or attend a sports event.

- If you are somewhere where there will be drinking, figure out what you're going to say ahead of time to anyone who offers a drink to you. Also, always take extra money and your cell phone to an event where your friends or other teens may be drinking. Never get into a car with someone who has been drinking.

- Call a taxi or your parents to come pick you up.

- If you're at a party with alcohol, drink something else instead, like soda or water.

You may have heard that drinking alcohol at a party helps you to loosen up, talk to people, and make new friends. But the truth is alcohol—no matter what amount—can make you have less control over what happens to you

☞ Remember!!

If someone is pressuring you to do anything that's not right or good for you, you have the right to resist. You have the right to say no, the right not to give a reason why, and the right to just walk away from a situation.

Resisting pressure can be hard for some people. Why?

- They are afraid of being rejected by others.

- They want to be liked and don't want to lose a friend.

- They don't want to be made fun of.

- They don't want to hurt someone's feelings.

- They aren't sure of what they really want.

- They don't know how to get out of the situation.

Sometimes resisting isn't easy, but you can do it with practice and a little know-how. Keep trying, even if you don't get it right at first.

Source: From "The Right To Resist," National Institute on Alcohol Abuse and Alcoholism (NIAAA), April 2006.

and your body. You can end up in uncomfortable or even dangerous situations. The best decision you can make is not to use alcohol at all. Most importantly, if you are drinking a soda or juice at a party, never put it down and go back to finish it. Someone can spike (put alcohol in) your drink or even put a drug in it.

Chapter 36

How To Help A Friend Who Has An Alcohol Problem

Step Up: What To Say

Discussing a friend's drug or alcohol use isn't an easy thing to do. It's very normal to worry about how a friend or sibling will respond to your concerns. If you're at a loss about how to start this type of discussion with someone you care about, we've compiled a list of steps, which may help with your approach and delivery.

Make A Plan

Before you engage your friend in a conversation, you'll need to prepare yourself. Go for a walk, sit where you can't be disturbed, and think. Reflect on the facts of the situation. Organize your thoughts. Decide what you want to say to your friend. Focus on a tone that is assertive, but not aggressive. Think about what resources you might need: a parent, a counselor, your faith leader, a school counselor, etc. Once you start the conversation, remain calm and supportive.

About This Chapter: This chapter includes information from "What To Say," an undated document produced by the Office of National Drug Control Policy; available at www.freevibe.com/stepup/whattosay.asp; accessed November 5, 2008.

Present The Facts

Discuss your concerns and identify some of the changes that you've seen in your friend. For example, you were at a party and saw your friend using drugs or acting in a way that you find inconsistent with their "normal" behavior; their grades have slipped or they're missing classes; your friend has changed from being "the person you know" to someone who is getting into trouble at home, or school, or in the community; or simply, you have noticed your friend has become quiet and secretive. Tell them you miss them and that you're concerned about them and that's why you want to talk. You may also decide that writing a note to your friend might be an appropriate first step.

Listen

After presenting your side of the story, ask your friend for his/her response to the information you've presented. Listen to your friend. Hear what he/she is saying. Offer your help, or ask them if they think they need a professional's help

Continue The Conversation

Determine a time when you and your friend will follow up about the discussion. Talking to your friend about drugs may be a continuous process—not a one-time event. Let your friend know that you'd like to touch base about the situation again in

---

✔ Quick Tip
Key Talking Points

- I don't want anything to happen to you or for you to hurt yourself.

- We all count on you. Your brothers/sisters (if applicable) look up to you/care about you, as do I. What would they do if you were gone? What would I do if you were gone?

- Look at all the things that you would miss out on. Drugs and alcohol can ruin your future and chances to keep your drivers' license, graduate, go to college, and get a job.

- What can I do to help you? I am here to support you.

- Are there other problems you want to talk about?

- Are you feeling pressure to use? Let's talk about it.

- I love you and I won't give up on you.

- If you need professional help or you need an adult to talk to, I can help you find someone. I will be here to help you and support you every step of the way.

the near future because you care about them. And, for you, don't be afraid to ask an adult who you can trust for help.

Talking To A Parent Or Supportive Adult

If you decide that your friend's problem is bigger than both of you, it may be time to bring the issue up with your parents, your friend's parents, or another supportive adult (coach, doctor, etc.). Keep in mind that only you know the people and relationships involved. Talking to a counselor about this decision may also be a good idea if you're not sure how your parents or your friend's parents will react.

It's Not Your Fault

Helping a friend with a drug or alcohol problem is hard work and can be a very difficult experience for you as well as your friend. You may feel a great

♣ It's A Fact!!

Sometimes, as much as you may try to get your friend to quit or seek help, you just can't seem to make it happen. If this becomes the situation you are in, you should do one of the following:

- Seek support from other friends or trusted adults—your friend is not the only one who needs help in this situation.

- Limit the time you spend with your drug or alcohol-using friend. Remember your friend's use may also be putting you at risk.

- Start thinking about yourself—get out and participate in activities that you enjoy to take your mind off of the situation.

deal of pressure to get your friend to stop drinking or doing drugs. Or you may get discouraged if your efforts to convince your friend to stop using drugs or alcohol don't work. But it is important to know that your friend's drug or alcohol use is not your fault. Remember that it's ultimately up to your friend to make that change and you can't do that for him.

Chapter 37

The Minimum Legal Drinking Age: Does It Help Prevent Alcohol-Related Problems?

Underage Drinking And The Minimum Legal Drinking Age

The extent and consequences of alcohol consumption by our nation's youth are matters of growing concern. Not only do most young people drink alcohol, but they often drink heavily, putting themselves and those around them at risk. The National Institute on Alcohol Abuse and Alcoholism (NIAAA) and other federal agencies continue to conduct and support research on how best to address underage drinking. In addition, adults in communities across the country are wrestling with how to change the culture around underage drinking. Although some have suggested that lowering the drinking age would lead to more responsible alcohol consumption among young people, the preponderance of research indicates that the legal drinking age of 21 has had positive effects on health and safety.

Laws Determine What Constitutes Underage Drinking

The Federal Uniform Drinking Age Act, signed into law in 1984, provides for withholding 10% of federal highway funds from states that do not

About This Chapter: This chapter includes "Research Findings on Underage Drinking and the Minimum Legal Drinking Age" and "Research Findings on College Drinking and the Minimum Legal Drinking Age." Both documents were produced by the National Institute on Alcohol Abuse and Alcoholism (NIAAA), October 2008.

prohibit the purchase or public possession of any alcoholic beverage by a person who is less than 21 years of age. This Act effectively raised the national minimum legal drinking age to 21, as all states ultimately complied. While it is illegal to sell alcohol to persons under 21 in all states, state laws vary widely with respect to specifics about possession and conditions under which consumption might be permissible (for example, with parents).

Negative Consequences Of Underage Drinking

In spite of these laws, we know underage drinking is widespread and is associated with a wide range of negative consequences.

The number of young people who drink and the way they drink results in harm to self and others including: risky sexual behavior; physical and sexual assaults; potential deleterious effects on the developing brain; problems in school, at work, and with the legal system; various types of injury; car crashes; homicide and suicide; and death from alcohol poisoning.

> ♣ **It's A Fact!!**
>
> Solving the problem of underage drinking will require a broad-based, long-term commitment. As we move forward, we need to pay attention to what history and research have taught us and build on this knowledge base including what we know about the relationship between minimum legal drinking age laws and underage drinking and its consequences.
>
> Source: "Research Findings on Underage Drinking and the Minimum Legal Drinking Age," NIAAA, October 2008.

Positive Effects Of Minimum Legal Drinking Age Laws

Minimum legal drinking age laws have had positive effects on health and safety. The preponderance of research shows minimum legal drinking age laws have had positive effects primarily in decreasing traffic crashes and fatalities, suicide, and decreased consumption by those under age 21.

Global Concerns

Minimum legal drinking ages vary by country but underage drinking is a problem around the world. While it has been suggested that lower legal drinking ages and different cultural norms in other countries (for example, France and Italy) may lead to better outcomes, survey data indicate this is generally not the case. Data from the 2003 European School Survey Project on Alcohol and Drugs (ESPAD) show that rates of binge drinking (five drinks or more in a row) and drunkenness among 15–16 year old students in the United States, France, and Italy are similar, with the United States lower on some measures and France and Italy lower on others.

College Drinking And The Minimum Legal Drinking Age

College drinking has been a frustratingly persistent problem on America's campuses. The tradition of drinking on and around campus is strong, and despite efforts to curtail the behavior, the majority of students—both under-age and of age—drink, many of them heavily. The negative consequences of alcohol consumption by our nation's college students are wide-ranging; they include academic problems, date rapes and assaults, and deaths from unintentional injuries and alcohol poisonings. Clearly, these consequences affect both drinkers and those around them.

Onset Of Drinking

For most, college drinking does not begin in college. Most students come to college having experienced alcohol in high school. By the 12th grade, 72 percent of high school students have had a full drink, 26 percent report engaging in binge drinking in the past two weeks, and 55 percent report ever having been drunk. Although colleges may "inherit" drinking problems, many students do increase their consumption when they get to college.

Culture Of Drinking

Drinking is deeply ingrained in the campus culture at many universities across the nation. Eighty-three percent of college students drink, and 41 percent report drinking five or more drinks on an occasion in the past two weeks, a particularly dangerous pattern of consumption. In addition, anecdotal reports and some research studies indicate that many college students drink far more than five drinks per occasion. An extreme example is the practice of attempting to drink 21 shots within the first hour starting at midnight of one's 21st birthday, which has resulted in alcohol poisonings.

The Prevalence Of High-Risk Drinking

Compared with all other age-groups, the prevalence of periodic heavy or high-risk drinking is greatest among young adults aged 18–24, whether they are in college, the military, or the workforce. In fact, the highest prevalence of alcohol dependence occurs in this age-group. Although college-bound 12th-graders are consistently less likely than their noncollege-bound counterparts to report occasions of heavy drinking, the higher rates of such drinking among college students compared with noncollege peers who entered the workforce indicate that college students catch up to and pass their working peers in binge drinking after high school graduation.

Problems Addressing College Drinking Patterns

Addressing college drinking is complicated by the fact that some student can drink legally, whereas others cannot. Whereas underage drinking laws apply only to drinking by individuals under age 21 and to those who provide alcohol to them, addressing the problem of excessive drinking for all students, not just those under 21, is critical to reducing alcohol-related consequences on and around campus. This combination of underage and of-age drinkers also is a problem for the military.

It is important to address college drinking both at the individual and the environmental level. Although there is no silver bullet, we do have evidence that a variety of individual, environmental, and campus–community approaches can work. Their effectiveness will depend on the culture and context of a particular campus. Generally, strategies that encompass multiple aspects of campus life, including the surrounding community, have been most successful. It also is important to note that underage drinking laws vary among states, and, therefore, college and university administrators need to understand how their state laws apply to their campuses.

Chapter 38

Deterring Alcohol-Impaired Drivers

Questions And Answers: Alcohol Deterrence And Enforcement

What is the goal of alcohol-impaired driving laws?

State laws making it illegal to drive with high blood alcohol concentrations (BACs) serve as the cornerstone of all efforts to reduce alcohol-impaired driving. Many people think the principal goal of such laws is to arrest and punish the drivers who put everyone else at risk. But arrest and punishment of offenders is a secondary objective. The most important objective is for the law to be a deterrent so that police find no alcohol-impaired drivers to arrest. This is commonly referred to as "general deterrence" because it targets and influences the general public. "Specific deterrence" refers to measures that seek to prevent re-offenses among individuals who have already committed an offense.

Why is deterrence so important and how can it be achieved?

Most impaired drivers are never stopped. Others are stopped, but police may miss signs of impairment. It was estimated that, in 1999, the chance of arrest when driving with a BAC at or above 0.08 percent was less than one in 50. Because the police cannot catch all offenders, the success of alcohol-impaired driving laws depends on deterring potential offenders by creating the public perception that apprehension and punishment is likely. Research has shown that the perceived likelihood of apprehension is more important in deterring offenders than the severity of punishment. The key to creating this perception is enforcement.

Merely putting strong laws on the books is not enough. Enforcement efforts must be sustained and well publicized to create a realistic threat of apprehension.

A variety of enforcement efforts are used to enforce alcohol-impaired driving laws. In some jurisdictions, specialized patrols work exclusively on

♣ It's A Fact!!
How do laws define alcohol-impaired driving?

The first state laws prohibited driving while intoxicated or while under the influence of alcohol. In practical terms, this meant that only obviously impaired drivers (so-called drunks) were likely to be arrested and, even then, it was difficult to obtain a conviction because no objective standard existed to prove intoxication. When the relationship between blood alcohol concentrations (BACs) and impairment of skills was established, it became possible to define offenses in terms of a BAC above a specific threshold.

Every state now uses BAC results to prosecute offenders. Initially, this was done through what are known as presumptive laws that establish a presumption of impairment at or above a specified BAC (defendants could try to rebut the presumption). All states and the District of Columbia have per se laws defining the offense as driving with a BAC above a prescribed limit, rather like a speed limit. Defendants can no longer try to prove they were not impaired, although they can challenge the validity of the BAC tests.

alcohol-impaired driving enforcement. Police in the majority of states can stop drivers at sobriety checkpoints. Sobriety checkpoints are one of the most effective approaches to deterring impaired driving.

Because there aren't enough police officers to apprehend all drivers impaired by alcohol, efforts to go beyond traditional enforcement and succeed in deterring potential offenders before they drive are ongoing. In almost all states, some alcohol impaired driving offenders are permitted to drive only if their vehicles have been equipped with alcohol ignition interlocks. These devices analyze a driver's breath and disable the ignition if the driver has been drinking. With funding from the federal government and motor vehicle manufacturers, an expert panel is overseeing the development of advanced in-vehicle alcohol detection technologies that would be suitable for all drivers, not just those convicted of alcohol-impaired driving. Challenges for the panel include addressing not only the devices' accuracy but also how quickly and unobtrusively they measure BACs. Institute research indicated that almost 9,000 deaths would have been prevented in 2005 if all drivers' BACs had been reduced to less than 0.08 percent.

What does blood alcohol concentration (BAC) measure?

A BAC describes the amount of alcohol in a person's blood, expressed as weight of alcohol per unit of volume of blood. For example, 0.08 percent BAC indicates 80 mg of alcohol per 100 ml of blood. For most legal purposes, however, a blood sample is not necessary to determine a person's BAC. It can be measured more simply by analyzing exhaled breath.

What is the BAC threshold for per se laws in the United States?

All 50 states and the District of Columbia have laws defining the BAC threshold as 0.08 percent.

How do BAC thresholds in the United States compare with those in other countries?

Alcohol-impaired driving is a serious problem throughout the industrialized world. BAC thresholds range from more than 0.08 percent in the United Kingdom to more than 0.05 percent in Australia and 0.02 percent or higher in Sweden. The European Commission, in 2001, recommended a blood alcohol limit not exceeding 0.05 percent for all drivers but novice and professional drivers who cannot exceed 0.02 percent. Among the 27 European Union member states, only Great Britain, Ireland, and Malta have BAC thresholds above 0.05 percent.

When can a driver be tested for alcohol in the U.S.?

In the United States, breath testing is considered a search, and the U.S. Constitution prohibits the searches unless the police have some reasonable basis for suspecting that a driver may be impaired by alcohol. U.S. police can carry out sobriety checkpoints that briefly stop some or all drivers, if the checkpoint is done in accordance with strict guidelines to ensure there is no discriminatory stopping of some people and not others. Even at a checkpoint, police must show they have a reasonable basis to administer a breath test to a driver. Depending on state law, police may be able to ask all drivers legally stopped to voluntarily consent to a breath test, but they cannot require a test without reasonable suspicion of an alcohol offense.

Other countries have different laws for testing drivers for alcohol. For example, in Australia police officers are allowed to administer a breath test to any driver, regardless of whether or not an officer has reason to believe the person has been drinking.

> ### ♣ It's A Fact!!
> ### How do sobriety checkpoints work?
>
> Police can use checkpoints to stop drivers at specified locations to identify impaired drivers. All drivers, or a predetermined proportion of them, are stopped based on rules that prevent police from arbitrarily selecting drivers to stop. Checkpoints are a visible enforcement method intended to deter potential offenders as well as to catch violators. If checkpoints are set up frequently over long enough periods and are well publicized, they can establish a convincing threat in people's minds that impaired drivers will be apprehended. This threat is key to general deterrence.
>
> In a survey of U.S. states conducted in 2002, thirty-seven states and the District of Columbia reported conducting checkpoints; thirteen reported not conducting them because of legal or policy reasons. Only 11 states reported conducting checkpoints as often as once a week.

Who can be stopped for alcohol-impaired driving?

Although police in the United States cannot stop and test individual drivers without cause, police can investigate any driver who, based on established criteria, appears to be driving while impaired by alcohol. Based on the totality of circumstances, they determine whether there is sufficient reason to detain the driver for an investigation of alcohol impairment. Although it is not required, many jurisdictions use a preliminary breath test (PBT), which is administered using a hand-held breath tester. After the officer makes an arrest, a court-admissible test is requested. In most states a driver can refuse this test, but refusal will result in license revocation or suspension.

Refusal rates vary greatly from state to state. A recent study found that refusal rates nationwide have remained stable at about one-quarter of all drivers arrested for alcohol-impaired driving from 1996 to 2001. California has the lowest refusal rate (five percent) and Rhode Island has the highest (85 percent). The consequences of refusal also vary by state. In some states, the administrative sanctions for a refusal are more stringent than those for failing a breath test. Some states have provisions to force a BAC test after a refusal.

Are sobriety checkpoints constitutional?

The U.S. Supreme Court held, in 1990, that properly conducted sobriety checkpoints are legal under the federal constitution. Most state courts that have addressed the issue have upheld checkpoints, too, but some have interpreted state law to prohibit checkpoints.

Which types of enforcement are most effective?

Measured in arrests per man-hour, a dedicated police patrol is the most effective method of apprehending offenders. Such patrols also may serve general deterrence if their activities are publicized and become widely known, but this usually is not the case. Sobriety checkpoints have been criticized for producing fewer arrests per man-hour than dedicated patrols, but some studies show arrest rates can be increased greatly when passive alcohol sensors are used to help police detect drinking drivers. In any case, focusing on the number of arrests is a misleading way to assess the value of checkpoints. The primary purpose of frequent checkpoints is to increase public awareness and deter potential offenders, resulting in the ideal situation of few offenders left to apprehend. For example, in the Australian state of Victoria, which has had an extensive roadside breath-testing program for several years, only one in 555 drivers stopped, in 1993, tested positive for alcohol to the point of breaking the law. In 1978, before the roadside breath-testing program, the ratio was one positive to 45 negatives.

A 1984 Institute study in two neighboring jurisdictions demonstrated how checkpoints can change public perceptions. Fairfax County, Virginia, had a long history of vigorous enforcement of alcohol-impaired driving laws and used unpublicized drinking-driver patrols to achieve relatively high arrest rates.

Nearby Montgomery County, Maryland had historically lower arrest rates but used well-publicized sobriety checkpoints during the study period. Surveys of licensed drivers revealed that public awareness of enforcement programs was far greater in Montgomery County than in Fairfax County. Respondents in both counties incorrectly believed the probability of arrest was higher in Montgomery County, where checkpoints were conducted.

These changed perceptions can lead to fewer crashes. Checkpoint programs in Florida, New Jersey, and Virginia have led to significant reductions in alcohol-related crashes. In 1988, the Institute and the city of Binghamton, New York implemented an integrated enforcement program that emphasized the publicized use of sobriety and safety belt checkpoints. During the program's first two years, the number of drivers stopped who had been drinking decreased about 40 percent. Late-night crashes decreased 21 percent while checkpoints were in place, and injury-producing nighttime crashes declined 16 percent. Results from North Carolina's 1995 statewide intensive three-week alcohol-impaired driving enforcement and publicity campaign indicated drivers with BACs at or above 0.08 percent declined from 198 per 10,000 before the program to 90 per 10,000 after.

In 2002, the Centers for Disease Control and Prevention reviewed studies in a variety of settings (urban, rural, and mixed) evaluating sobriety checkpoint programs. The median decline in fatal crashes thought to involve alcohol was about 20 percent.

Low-manpower checkpoints with as few as three to five officers can be effective in reducing the percentage of drivers operating at higher BACs. Institute research found that police agencies in two rural counties in West Virginia were able to sustain a yearlong program of weekly low-manpower checkpoints. The proportion of nighttime drivers with BACs at or above 0.05 percent was 70 percent lower following implementation of the checkpoint program, compared with drivers in other counties where additional checkpoints were not conducted.

♣ It's A Fact!!
If sobriety checkpoints are so effective, why aren't they more widely used?

In 10 states, sobriety checkpoints cannot be conducted because they are illegal under these states' constitutions or statutes. In other states, sobriety checkpoints may be underutilized because police departments believe a large number of officers are required, placing checkpoints beyond the resources of small police agencies and draining the personnel and financial resources of larger agencies. However, research by the Institute and others has shown that small-scale checkpoints with only a few officers can be conducted successfully and safely and can be effective in reducing alcohol-impaired driving and alcohol-related crashes. The federal government encourages states to do frequent, low-manpower checkpoints, which can be conducted with three to five officers.

How can passive alcohol sensors aid in enforcement?

Many people can effectively mask the overt behavioral symptoms of alcohol impairment for short periods, but it is much more difficult to hide the evidence of impairment from a passive alcohol sensor, which identifies alcohol in the exhaled breath near a driver's mouth. Passive alcohol sensors are screening devices that help an officer detect possible impaired drivers for further testing. The sensors are not intrusive and therefore do not violate constitutional prohibitions against unreasonable search and seizure. In a 1993

Institute study of sobriety checkpoints in Fairfax County, Virginia police officers using sensors were able to detect more offenders compared with officers who did not use sensors. Police without sensors detected 55 percent of drivers whose BACs were at or above 0.10 percent. With sensors, police successfully detected 71 percent of the drivers with BACs at or above 0.10 percent. Results of the Fairfax study parallel previous Institute evaluations.

Is license suspension an effective sanction?

Laws providing for the suspension or revocation of licenses have been shown to reduce the subsequent crash involvement of drivers convicted of alcohol offenses. Even after the suspension, the effects last. Although many suspended drivers continue to drive, they tend to drive less. License suspension also has led to a general reduction in fatal crashes in states where the threat of this sanction has been made more certain through laws that provide for administrative license suspension.

Would more severe sanctions reduce the problem?

The surprising answer is, probably not. Sanctions range from fines and license suspension to jail terms or community service. Historically, the potential punishment has been severe. However, the probability of apprehension has been low and some penalties infrequently applied even if mandatory by statute. In fact, a sanction may be more likely to be applied when judges and juries consider it to be appropriate but not too severe, such as license suspension.

The world's first per se drinking driving laws, enacted in Norway in 1936 and Sweden in 1941, were regarded as strict because imprisonment routinely was imposed on drivers apprehended with high BACs. However, a 1975 evaluation of the effects of these laws showed no significant change in the number or rate of fatal motor vehicle crashes. The notion that the sanctions were effective has thus been characterized as "the Scandinavian myth."

What is the effect of treatment and rehabilitation programs?

Although studies have had mixed results, research has shown that treatment and rehabilitation programs may have a small, positive effect on the subsequent behavior of alcohol-impaired driving offenders. Several evaluations of 35 alcohol and treatment programs (Alcohol Safety Action Projects), implemented in the 1970s, found lower re-offense rates for first offenders compared with repeat offenders, but no effect on crash rates. A 1995 examination of more than 200 studies of the effects of various treatment and rehabilitation programs found a reduction of seven to nine percent, on average, in subsequent alcohol-impaired driving events including both alcohol-impaired driving re-offenses and alcohol-involved crashes. A 1997 study of California programs found that treatment combined with driver license penalties was more effective than license penalties alone in reducing repeat offenses among first and repeat offenders. Treatment and rehabilitation in lieu of license sanctions or other penalties have not been shown effective in reducing recidivism or alcohol-involved crashes.

Which laws have been most effective in the United States?

In a 1989 study, Institute researchers evaluated the effectiveness of administrative license suspension laws, per se BAC laws, and laws requiring jail or community service after a first alcohol-impaired driving offense. During the mostly late-night hours when at least half of all fatally injured drivers had BACs at or above 0.10 percent, administrative license suspension laws were estimated to reduce driver involvement in fatal crashes by about nine percent. Laws requiring jail or community service for a first offense were estimated to reduce driver involvement in fatal crashes by about six percent. The effect of per se BAC laws was an estimated six percent reduction in crash involvement during daytime hours when fatal crashes typically are less likely to involve alcohol. A review by the Centers for Disease Control and Prevention of the effects of lowering per se BAC thresholds from 0.10 to 0.08 percent found a median decrease of seven percent in alcohol-related motor vehicle fatalities.

Have other countries done a better job controlling alcohol-impaired driving?

In many countries around the world, including the United States, substantial progress against alcohol-impaired driving was achieved from the early 1980s through the mid 1990s. In recent years, substantial reductions in deaths related to driving under the influence of alcohol have been achieved in some European countries. From 1996–1998 to 2005, Germany, the Netherlands, and the Czech Republic reduced drunk-driving deaths by 50 percent. However, this is not the case for all European countries. In Great Britain, Spain, Finland, Lithuania, and Hungary, the average yearly percentage change in alcohol-related crash deaths increased slightly and some other European countries do not even keep track of alcohol-related crashes.

Australia has the most successful documented programs to reduce alcohol-impaired driving. All programs have in common highly visible, sustained, widespread enforcement. The state of Victoria maintains an aggressive program of random breath testing of drivers. The percentage of drivers and motorcyclists killed in crashes with BACs above 0.05 percent dropped from 50 percent in 1977 to about 25 percent in 1995, indicating the deterrent result of a long-term, high-visibility enforcement program.

> ✤ **It's A Fact!!**
>
> Laws establishing a minimum age for purchasing alcohol also have proved effective in reducing nighttime fatal crashes among young drivers. An Institute study conducted in 26 states that raised the minimum legal purchase ages during 1975–84 estimated a 13 percent reduction in nighttime driver fatal crash involvement. Zero tolerance laws that set zero BAC thresholds for drivers younger than 21 also have been shown to reduce crashes likely to involve alcohol impairment among drivers ages 15–20.

Do alcohol ignition interlocks have a role in deterrence?

Yes, studies have shown alcohol ignition interlocks to be effective in reducing recidivism among persons convicted of alcohol-impaired driving.

An alcohol ignition interlock has a breath-testing unit that is connected to a vehicle's ignition. In order to start the vehicle, the driver must blow into the device and register a blood alcohol reading that is below a pre-determined level. If the blood alcohol reading exceeds this level, the interlock prevents the vehicle from starting.

In a 1999 Institute study, multiple offenders eligible for license reinstatement were randomly assigned to participate in an ignition interlock program or the conventional postlicensing treatment program. Participation in the interlock program reduced the risk of committing an alcohol-related traffic violation within the first year following conviction by nearly 65 percent. Other studies also have found lower recidivism rates when an interlock device is installed on a vehicle, but any benefits disappear when the device is removed.

Two states (New Mexico and Arizona) require as a condition of relicensing all eligible first offenders to equip their vehicles with ignition interlocks following conviction. Most states allow or require ignition interlocks for at least some repeat offenders, and some states' laws also apply to first offenders with very high BACs (for example, at or above 0.15 percent). However, studies of these laws have found very low participation rates. In a 2007 study in New Mexico, researchers found that of the over 21,000 repeat offenders eligible for interlocks, less than five percent installed one. Similarly, a 2002 study of California's interlock program found that despite a mandatory requirement of interlocks for drivers convicted of alcohol-impaired driving while on a driving under the influence-suspended (DUI-suspended) license, less than 10 percent had a device installed. As of 2006, there were an estimated 100,000 interlocks in use in the United States representing only a tiny portion of the approximately 1.4 million annual driving while intoxicated (DWI) convictions for alcohol-impaired driving.

♣ **It's A Fact!!**

A cooperative venture of motor vehicle manufacturers and the federal government is overseeing the development of advanced in-vehicle alcohol detection technologies that would be suitable for all drivers, not just convicted offenders. The goal is to develop a device that can quickly, accurately, and unobtrusively measure blood alcohol concentrations (BACs).

Part Six
Children Of Alcoholics

Chapter 39

Families With A History Of Alcohol Dependence

If you are among the millions of people in this country who have a parent, grandparent, or other close relative with alcoholism, you may have wondered what your family's history of alcoholism means for you. Are problems with alcohol a part of your future? Is your risk for becoming an alcoholic greater than for people who do not have a family history of alcoholism? If so, what can you do to lower your risk?

Many scientific studies, including research conducted among twins and have shown that genetic factors influence alcoholism. These findings show that children of alcoholics are general population to develop alcohol problems. Children of alcoholics also have a higher risk for many other behavioral and emotional problems. But alcoholism is not determined only by the genes you inherit from your parents. In fact, more than one-half of all children of alcoholics do not become alcoholic. Research shows that many factors influence your risk of developing alcoholism. Some factors raise the risk while others lower it.

Genes are not the only things children inherit from their parents. How parents act and how they treat each other and their children has an influence

About This Chapter: This chapter includes information from "A Family History Of Alcoholism: Are You At Risk?" National Institute on Alcohol Abuse and Alcoholism (NIAAA), February 2003. The information in this chapter was reviewed for currency by David A. Cooke, M.D., in December 2008.

on children growing up in the family. These aspects of family life also affect the risk for alcoholism. Researchers believe a person's risk increases if he or she is in a family with difficulties, such as those listed below.

- An alcoholic parent is depressed or has other psychological problems

- Both parents abuse alcohol and other drugs

- The parents' alcohol abuse is severe

- Conflicts lead to aggression and violence in the family

The good news is that many children of alcoholics from even the most troubled families do not develop drinking problems. Just as a family history of alcoholism does not guarantee that you will become an alcoholic, neither does growing up in a very troubled household with alcoholic parents. Just because alcoholism tends to run in families does not mean that a child of an alcoholic parent will automatically become an alcoholic too. The risk is higher but it does not have to happen.

> ♣ **It's A Fact!!**
>
> - Approximately 17.6 million American adults abuse alcohol or are alcohol dependent
>
> - Approximately one in four children is exposed to effects of alcohol abuse or dependence in a family member
>
> Source: "Alcohol And The Family," National Institute on Alcohol Abuse and Alcoholism (NIAAA), August 2004.

> ♣ **It's A Fact!!**
>
> Exposure to a parent's alcohol use disorder may result in easy access to alcohol by children, adolescents, and young adults; establish norms of tolerating heavy alcohol use by family members; result in poor/absent parental monitoring of alcohol use by children, adolescents, young adults; and lead to development of risky "alcohol expectancies" early in life. Parenting practices can also be affected by alcohol use disorders.
>
> - Family life may be chaotic and involve poor quality environments
>
> - Children's exposure to conflict is common
>
> Source: "Alcohol And The Family," National Institute on Alcohol Abuse and Alcoholism (NIAAA), August 2004.

If you are worried that your family's history of alcohol problems or your troubled family life puts you at risk for becoming alcoholic, here is some common-sense advice to help you.

Avoid underage drinking: First, underage drinking is illegal. Second, research shows that the risk for alcoholism is higher among people who begin to drink at an early age, perhaps as a result of both environmental and genetic factors.

Drink moderately as an adult: Even if they do not have a family history of alcoholism, adults who choose to drink alcohol should do so in moderation—no more than one drink a day for most women, and no more than two drinks a day for most men, according to guidelines from the U.S. Department of Agriculture and the U.S. Department of Health and Human Services. Some people should not drink at all, including women who are pregnant or who are trying to become pregnant, recovering alcoholics, people who plan to drive or engage in other activities that require attention or skill, people taking certain medications, and people with certain medical conditions.

People with a family history of alcoholism, who have a higher risk for becoming dependent on alcohol, should approach moderate drinking carefully. Maintaining moderate drinking habits may be harder for them than for people without a family history of drinking problems. Once a person moves from moderate to heavier drinking, the risks of

♣ It's A Fact!!

Family is relevant because alcohol may influence family functioning; family functioning affects alcohol use/abuse; and alcohol use disorders run in families. Families can take many diverse forms.

- Nuclear

- Single parent mother

- Single parent father

- Ex-and step-relations

- Grandparent, aunt/uncle as parent

- Foster families

- And others

Source: "Alcohol And The Family," National Institute on Alcohol Abuse and Alcoholism (NIAAA), August 2004.

> ♣ **It's A Fact!!**
>
> Children from families of alcoholics are at increased risk for alcohol dependence throughout their lives. More than three decades of research has firmly established that genes account for over half of the risk for alcohol dependence, and environmental factors account for the remainder. Researchers have succeeded in identifying regions of chromosomes associated with an altered risk of developing alcohol dependence and, in some cases, individual genes and candidate genes but no single gene that accounts for the majority of risk. The development of a complex behavioral disorder such as alcohol dependence likely depends on specific genetic factors interacting with one another, multiple environmental factors, and the interaction between genetic and environmental factors. Important when considering underage drinking is research suggesting that genes have a stronger influence over the development of problem use, whereas environment seems to play a greater role in the initiation of alcohol use.
>
> Source: "Adolescents from Families with a History of Alcohol Dependence," from *The Surgeon General's Call To Action To Prevent And Reduce Underage Drinking*, Office of the Surgeon General, U.S. Department of Health and Human Services, 2007.

social problems (for example, drinking and driving, violence, and trauma) and medical problems (for example, liver disease, brain damage, and cancer) increase greatly.

Talk to a health care professional: Discuss your concerns with a doctor, nurse, nurse practitioner, or other health care provider. They can recommend groups or organizations that could help you avoid alcohol problems. If you are an adult who already has begun to drink, a health care professional can assess your drinking habits to see if you need to cut back on your drinking and advise you about how to do that.

Chapter 40

Alcoholism Tends To Run In Families

Children Of Alcoholics

Alcoholism and other drug addiction tend to run in families. Children of addicted parents are more at risk for alcoholism and other drug abuse than are other children.

- Children of addicted parents are the group of children most at risk of becoming alcohol and drug abusers due to both genetic and family environment factors.

- Children with a biological parent who is alcoholic continue to have an increased risk (two to ninefold) of developing alcoholism even when they have been adopted. This fact supports the hypothesis that there is a genetic component in alcoholism.

- Recent studies further suggest a strong genetic component, particularly for early onset of alcoholism in males. Sons of alcoholic fathers

About This Chapter: This chapter begins with information from "Children of Alcoholics: A Kit For Educators," © 2001 National Association for Children of Alcoholics (www.nacoa.net). Reprinted with permission. To view the complete text of this booklet including references, visit http://www.nacoa.net/pdfs/EDkit_web_06.pdf. Additional information is excerpted from "Alcoholism Tends to Run in Families," Substance Abuse and Mental Health Services Administration (SAMHSA), 1995. The information in this chapter was reviewed for currency by David A. Cooke, M.D., in December 2008.

are at fourfold risk (of future substance abuse) compared with the male offspring of non-alcoholic fathers.

• Use of substances by parents and their adolescent children is strongly correlated; generally, if parents take drugs, sooner or later their children will also. Adolescents who use drugs are more likely than their non-addicted peers to have one or more parents who also use drugs.

Family interaction is defined by substance abuse or addiction in a family.

• Families affected by alcoholism report higher levels of conflict than do families with no alcoholism. Drinking is the primary factor in family disruption. The environment of children of alcoholics has been characterized by lack of parenting, poor home management, and lack of family communication skills, thereby effectively robbing children of alcoholic parents of modeling or training in parenting skills or family effectiveness.

> **♣ It's A Fact!!**
>
> The influence of parental attitudes on a child's drug-taking behaviors may be as important as actual drug abuse by the parents. An adolescent who perceives that a parent is permissive about the use of drugs is more likely to use drugs.
>
> Source: © 2001 National Association for Children of Alcoholics.

• The following family problems have frequently been associated with families affected by alcoholism: increased family conflict; emotional or physical violence; decreased family cohesion; decreased family organization; increased family isolation; increased family stress including work problems, illness, marital strain and financial problems; and frequent family moves.

• Addicted parents often lack the ability to provide structure or discipline in family life, but simultaneously expect their children to be competent at a wide variety of tasks earlier than do non-addicted parents.

• Sons of addicted fathers are the recipients of more detrimental discipline practices from their parents.

A relationship between parental addiction and child abuse is indicated in a large proportion of child abuse and neglect cases.

- Three of four (71.6%) child welfare professionals cite substance abuse as the chief cause for the dramatic rise in child maltreatment since 1986.

- Most welfare professionals (79.6%) report that substance abuse causes or contributes to at least half of all cases of child maltreatment; 39.7% say it is a factor in over 75% of the cases.

- In a sample of parents who significantly maltreat their children, alcohol abuse specifically is associated with physical maltreatment, while cocaine abuse exhibits a specific relationship to sexual maltreatment.

- Children exposed prenatally to illicit drugs are two to three times more likely to be abused or neglected.

Children of drug addicted parents are at greater risk for placement outside the home.

- Three of four child welfare professionals (75.7%) say that children of addicted parents are more likely to enter foster care, and 73% say that children of alcoholics stay longer in foster care than do other children.

- In one study, 79% of adolescent runaways and homeless youth reported alcohol use in the home, 53% reported problem drinking in the home, and 54% reported drug use in the home.

- Each year, approximately 11,900 infants are abandoned at birth or are kept at hospitals, 78% of whom are drug-exposed. The average daily cost for each of these babies is $460.

Children of addicted parents exhibit symptoms of depression and anxiety more than do children from non-addicted families.

- Children of addicted parents exhibit depression and depressive symptoms more frequently than do children from non-addicted families.

- Children of addicted parents are more likely to have anxiety disorders or to show anxiety symptoms.

- Children of addicted parents are at high risk for elevated rates of psychiatric and psychosocial dysfunction, as well as for alcoholism.

Children of addicted parents experience greater physical and mental health problems and generate higher health and welfare costs than do children from non-addicted families.

- Inpatient admission rates and average lengths of stay for children of alcoholics are 25–30% greater than for children of non-alcoholic parents. Substance abuse and other mental disorders are the most notable conditions among children of addiction.

- It is estimated that parental substance abuse and addiction are the chief cause in 70–90% of all child welfare spending. Using the more conservative 70% assessment, in 1998 substance abuse and addiction accounted for approximately $10 billion in federal, state and local government spending simply to maintain child welfare systems.

- The economic costs associated with fetal alcohol syndrome were estimated at $1.9 billion for 1992.

- A sample of children hospitalized for psychiatric disorders demonstrated that more than 50% were children of addicted parents.

Children of addicted parents have a higher-than-average rate of behavior problems.

- One study comparing children of alcoholics (aged 6–17 years) with children of psychiatrically healthy medical patients, found that children of alcoholics had elevated rates of ADHD (attention deficit hyperactivity disorder) and ODD (oppositional defiant disorder) compared to the control group of children.

- Research on behavioral problems demonstrated by children of alcoholics has revealed some of the following traits: lack of empathy for other persons, decreased social adequacy and interpersonal adaptability, low self-esteem, and lack of control over the environment.

- Research has shown that children of addicted parents demonstrate behavioral characteristics and a temperament style that predispose them to future maladjustment.

Children of addicted parents score lower on tests measuring school achievement and exhibit other difficulties in school.

- Sons of addicted parents performed worse on all domains measuring school achievement, using the Peabody Individual Achievement Test-Revised (PIAT-R), including general information, reading recognition, reading comprehension, total reading, mathematics, and spelling.

- In general, children of alcoholic parents do less well on academic measures. They also have higher rates of school absenteeism and are more likely to leave school, be retained, or be referred to the school psychologist than are children of non-alcoholic parents.

- In one study, 41% of addicted parents reported that at least one of their children repeated a grade in school, 19% were involved in truancy, and 30% had been suspended from school.

- Children of addicted parents were found at significant disadvantage on standard scores of arithmetic compared to children of non-addicted parents.

✤ It's A Fact!!

Children of alcoholic parents often believe that they will be failures even if they do well academically. They often do not view themselves as successful.

Source: © 2001 National Association for Children of Alcoholics.

Children of addicted parents score lower on tests measuring verbal ability.

- Children of addicted parents tend to score lower on tests that measure cognitive and verbal skills.

- Their ability to express themselves may be impaired, which can hamper their school performance, peer relationships, ability to develop and sustain intimate relationships, and performance on job interviews.

- Lower verbal scores, however, should not imply that children of addicted parents are intellectually impaired.

Children of addicted parents have greater difficulty with abstraction and conceptual reasoning.

- Abstraction and conceptual reasoning play an important role in problem solving, whether the problems are academic or are related to situations encountered in life. Children of alcoholics may require very concrete explanations and instructions.

Maternal consumption of alcohol and other drugs any time during pregnancy can cause birth defects or neurological deficits.

- Studies have shown that exposure to cocaine during fetal development may lead to subtle but significant deficits later on, especially with skills that are crucial to success in the classroom, such as the ability to block distractions and concentrate for long periods.

- Cognitive performance is less affected by alcohol exposure in infants and children whose mothers stopped drinking in early pregnancy, despite the mothers' resumption of alcohol use after giving birth.

♣ It's A Fact!!

Children of addicted parents may benefit from supportive adult efforts to help them.

- Children who coped effectively with the trauma of growing up in families affected by alcoholism often relied on the support of a non-alcoholic parent, step-parent, grandparent, teachers and others.

- Children in families affected by addiction who can rely on other supportive adults have greater autonomy and independence, stronger social skills, better ability to cope with difficult emotional experiences, and better day-to-day coping strategies than other children of addicted parents.

- Group programs reduce feelings of isolation, shame and guilt among children of alcoholics while capitalizing on the importance to adolescents of peer influence and mutual support.

- Competencies such as the ability to establish and maintain intimate relationships, express feelings, and solve problems can be improved by building the self-esteem and self-efficacy of children of alcoholics.

Source: © 2001 National Association for Children of Alcoholics.

- Prenatal alcohol effects have been detected at moderate levels of alcohol consumption in nonalcoholic women. Even though a mother may not regularly abuse alcohol, her child may not be spared the effects of prenatal alcohol exposure.

Alcoholism Tends To Run In Families

What's important about children of alcoholics?

Children of alcoholics (COAs) are at high risk for alcohol and other drug problems; often live with pervasive tension and stress; have higher levels of anxiety and depression; do poorly in school; and experience problems with coping. The good news is that they can be helped to bounce back from the effects of their families' problems.

When family members (parents, grandparents, aunts/uncles), guardians, or other adults in charge of children are alcoholics, there is strong evidence that children in these families are more likely to develop the disease of alcoholism as well. The fact is, alcoholism tends to run in families.

What causes COAs to have increased risk?

Children of alcoholics may or may not be raised by alcoholics. Either way, every COA is at risk for alcoholism or alcoholism-related problems.

- **Children Living With Alcoholics:** Children who live with alcoholics are at increased risk because of genetic and/or environmental factors. They may be at more risk for alcoholism just as children of diabetics are at higher risk for diabetes. Children living with alcoholics often develop unhealthy living patterns. They may not learn how to trust themselves or others, how to handle uncomfortable feelings, or how to build positive relationships. COAs who lack these skills are also at higher risk for school failure, depression, increased anxiety, as well as trouble with alcohol and other drugs.

- **Adopted And Foster Children:** Even COAs adopted by non-alcoholics (or do not live with their alcoholic parents for other reasons), may have a genetic predisposition to alcoholism, just as children born to parents with a history of heart disease are more at risk for heart disease.

Alcoholism can skip a generation. Some COAs never drink, but may pass on a genetic vulnerability and/or unhealthy living pattern to their own children.

COAs do not have to develop problems. Genes can't be replaced. But unhealthy living patterns can be countered by the consistent caring of others. COAs can learn to trust, handle their feelings in healthy ways, and build positive, nurturing relationships. Anyone can help COAs understand their risks and learn better social and coping skills.

How many COAs are there? How many become alcoholics?

There were an estimated 28.6 million COAs in the U.S. in 1991, nearly 11 million of them under age 18. Of the under-18 group, almost three million will develop alcoholism, other drug problems, and/or other serious coping problems. About half of COAs marry alcoholics and are likely to recreate the same kinds of highly stressful and unhealthy families in which they grew up, unless supportive interventions are provided to them in their formative years.

♣ It's A Fact!!

Even children of alcoholics (COAs) in high-risk environments with other chronic sources of stress—including poverty, racism, disrupted marriages, serious emotional problems, and histories of abuse and neglect—are often able to overcome these painful beginnings and create healthy, fulfilling lives for themselves.

Source: SAMHSA, 1995.

What about the other COAs?

Based on stories from adult COAs in professional treatment and self-help programs, it appears all children are affected by family alcoholism. But, going back to the good news, many of them make positive adjustments to their families' alcoholism.

How can COAs be helped to "bounce back?"

This is where the good news is really exciting. The child in an alcoholic home may be helped whether the alcoholic stops drinking or not. It is not necessary to do anything to change the adult's drinking behavior. And helping a COA does not require special training or skills.

✔ Quick Tip
More Things To Do

Follow through if someone asks for help, because it probably required a lot of courage for her/him
to do so. Know the local number for Alateen and other
sources of help you can offer as needed. Let them know they
aren't alone; there are approximately 11 million COAs under the
age of 18. Collect information about alcoholism to discuss with the
child when it's comfortable for both of you to do so. Be aware and re-
spectful of cultural differences, such as family structure, customs, values,
and beliefs. Be aware that some COAs may have been mistreated and
may be threatened by displays of affection, especially physical contact. Help them make discoveries, positive connections; instill
enthusiasm for life and all its many possibilities.

And, when talking with anyone under 21 about
alcohol and other drugs, urge them to "Be smart.
Don't start."

Source: SAMHSA, 1995.

Simple acts of kindness and compassion can make a big difference in the lives of COAs. Just by "being there," to lend an ear, share normal interests and activities, talk about feelings, accept their mistakes, and support and encourage their friend-making efforts, you will be helping.

What else helps COAs?

Tell them that they did not cause alcoholism and cannot cure or control it. But they can learn to cope with it. Make clear that children are not re-sponsible for solving grown-up problems.

Understand that COAs often build up defenses against the pain, shame, guilt, or loneliness they may feel. They may show off, act tough, keep secrets, or hide. You may help by just accepting them for who they are. Encouraging them to share their thoughts and feelings will help them learn to trust others and accept and adjust to their lives.

Get them involved in something about which they feel good. It can be something small like taking care of a pet; or a hobby such as collecting rocks, or stamps, or comic books; or a sport. Go slow, don't push, but keep trying.

Gently help them get positive attention from others. Let them know they are wonderful, special, and cared about just because they are who they are. Again, go slowly, but tell them often.

Help them see life as really living even though there are times and situations that may be very painful. Help them see beyond their present circumstances. Help them feel connected to nature, art, and history; to heritage, culture, religion; and to their community. Help them build a larger picture of their lives and their world than their families' current problems.

Help them understand that it is okay to ask for help. Assure them that getting help is a sign of strength. Offer some examples from your own life so they'll know how it's done and that it really is okay.

Chapter 41

Understanding The Alcoholic Family

Family Values

It's sometimes called the "three-generation" disease, passed from parent to children to grandchildren, like red hair or freckles.

But it's way more serious than that, and it doesn't seem to be going away.

According to the best estimates, about one in eight Americans—more than 30 million of us—are products of alcoholic homes. And the National Institute on Alcohol Abuse and Alcoholism says that 6.6 million kids are living with an alcoholic parent right now.

What's life like for them?

Well, it doesn't look like the families in Norman Rockwell paintings or feel much like the Baileys in *It's a Wonderful Life*.

More often, it's like an endless marathon of *Married with Children* episodes, where growing up is a constant struggle to cope with disappointment and stress and embarrassment.

About This Chapter: This chapter includes information from "Children Of Alcoholics: How To Help When A Parent Has A Problem," © 2007 Do It Now Foundation (www.doitnow.org). Reprinted with permission.

It's a place where a kid's needs are often down-played or ignored, and family life centers on the psychological "games" of the drinking parent. Consider:

- Fifty-five percent of all family violence occurs in alcoholic homes.

- Incest is twice as likely among daughters of alcoholics than their peers.

- Children of alcoholics are three to four times more likely to become alcoholic than the general population.

- Fifty percent of children of alcoholics marry an alcoholic; 70 percent develop a pattern of compulsive behavior as an adult, including alcoholism, drug abuse, and overeating.

And no statistic can measure the psychological pain that children of alcoholics grow up with and often carry into adulthood.

Until recently, children of alcoholics weren't even considered all that different from other kids with problems. Often, they were ignored by treatment programs, which focused on the alcoholic parent.

Now that's changing. Today, professionals recognize the special problems and needs of children of alcoholics (or COAs), and family therapy has become a big part of alcoholism rehabilitation.

And treating the problem—rebuilding self-esteem and relearning to communicate and trust and love—begins with identifying what, exactly, went wrong in the first place.

The Alcoholic Family

One reason identifying children of alcoholics can be so difficult is that many kids—maybe even most kids—don't like to admit that there are troubles at home.

That's because denial can play as big a role in the life of an alcoholic family as it does in the process of alcoholism itself. When a drinking parent denies that drinking is a problem, kids usually learn pretty fast that one thing that's virtually guaranteed to cause upset is for them to talk about it—or even think about it much, at all.

The conflict that comes from denying the obvious and the struggle to keep up appearances for outsiders can trigger emotional tremors for COAs that can reverberate for years.

Common problems can include:

- **Guilt:** The child suspects that he or she somehow caused the parent's drinking.

- **Anxiety:** Fear of arguments or violence can cause constant worry and emotional hypervigilance.

- **Embarrassment:** The child is ashamed of the family "secret" and withdraws from friends or other family members.

- **Confusion:** A drinking parent's mood swings and unpredictability can cause uncertainty and inner turmoil in the child about what to do next.

- **Inability To Trust:** Repeated disappointments and broken promises by an alcoholic parent can make it hard for a child to trust and develop close bonds with others.

- **Anger:** The child usually resents the drinking parent and may transfer the anger to the non-drinking parent for lack of support and protection.

- **Depression:** Feelings of loneliness and helplessness are common—and almost inevitable.

In an alcoholic family, a child's need for love, support, and emotional nurturing is often minimized or forgotten altogether in the endless tug-of-war between the family and alcoholism.

And with few role models for demonstrating how emotions can be expressed positively, the child adapts to chaos in order to survive.

The Family Drama

The constant hurt and confusion of the alcoholic household often reveals itself in children protecting themselves by lying, suppressing feelings, and withdrawing from close relationships.

♣ It's A Fact!!
If Your Mom Or Dad Drinks Too Much

Some of the things we've talked about in this chapter may sound familiar. In fact, if one of your parents is an active alcoholic, it may describe what's going on in your family right now. If that's the case, you're due for some good news, and here it is: There are things you can do to help clear up the problem.

- **Step 1:** The first thing to do is to realize that you aren't alone. Millions of kids have been through the same problem and have felt the same fears. These kids (many of them adults now) have been where you are and know what you're feeling, and they know how to help.

- **Step 2:** The next thing to do is to tell someone. If you have a cool teacher or friend or a favorite aunt or uncle, talk with them and don't hold back. Even though it might seem easier and safer to keep things a secret, what really hurts you over the long term is keeping problems stuffed inside yourself. Others understand and they can help.

- **Step 3:** The last thing to do if you're the child of an alcoholic is to realize that it's not your fault. Your parents may love you, but your parents have a problem. The best way you can help them is to help yourself. Call a local Al-Anon or AlaTeen chapter (they're listed in the white pages of the phone book) or write the Children of Alcoholics Foundation, 540 Madison Avenue, New York, NY 10022. For immediate referral to services in your area, call the Boys Town National Hotline at 1-800-448-3000.

And do it now. Drinking or drugs may be your family's problem today, but they don't have to be a problem forever.

Having learned these defenses in adolescence, children of alcoholics tend to repeat them in adulthood, usually without realizing the connection.

One leading therapist, Dr. Claudia Black, says that children from alcoholic homes tend to adopt a distinct role within the family.

Dr. Black, a COA herself and national advocate for children's rights, cites four common roles that recur in alcoholic households:

- **Responsible Child:** Some kids assume the role of the parent by feeding and caring for younger brothers and sisters.

- **Adjuster Child:** Here, kids simply accept whatever behavior a drinking parent dishes out. Many hide and become quiet and withdrawn.

- **Acting-Out Child:** Some children assume blame for their parent's drinking and deflect attention from family problems by creating problems of their own at home and school.

- **Placater Child:** These kids ignore their own unhappiness to comfort others. Some become family clowns and try to cover problems with jokes.

According to Dr. Black, children of alcoholics can become such experts at playing their roles that they often create situations as adults where they continue to act out the family drama. This strong role identification, she argues, is one reason that many adult children of alcoholics marry problem drinkers.

The Healing Process

Probably the most difficult step in the healing process is the first one—for the child to openly identify the problem and begin to talk about his or her sadness and anger. Out of love or fear, most children try to keep family problems a secret.

Believing that they're the ones with the problem and may even be somehow to blame, children with drinking parents often hide behind a wall of denial and defensiveness.

Identifying a child of an alcoholic usually involves little more than close observation of changes or extremes in the child's behavior.

A number of behavioral signs can warn of a parental drinking problem, including:

- School absences or truancy

- Withdrawal from classmates and friends

- Frequent illness or physical complaints

- Drug or alcohol abuse

- Overly aggressive play

- Delinquent behavior

- Under-achievement in school

- Emotional distance from peers

✤ It's A Fact!!

Bouncing Back: Reasons And Resources

Problem drinking touches more lives—and wrecks more families—than you might think.

According to a recent study by the U.S. Department of Health and Human Services:

- Seventy-six million Americans (43 percent of the adult population) report alcoholism in their families.

- Eighteen percent say they grew up with an alcoholic or problem drinker.

- Thirty-eight percent of U.S. adults have at least one blood relative with a drinking problem.

And the problem doesn't end with simple drinking. Physical and sexual abuse are both linked to problem drinking, as are higher rates of divorce, homicide, and suicide.

What's the solution? There are a lot of different solutions, according to experts, and they all begin with those affected taking responsibility for ending the problem.

If problem drinking is a problem for you or someone you care about, do something to stop it now. Contact the National Council on Alcoholism and Drug Dependence at 1-800-622-2255 or a local chapter of Alcoholics Anonymous (check the White Pages of your phone book).

And do it now. Problem drinking is a problem that's wasted too many lives for too long.

Once a child of an alcoholic is identified and begins to confront his or her suppressed guilt and fears, the real process of recovery can begin.

Since learning about the dynamics of alcoholism is important to the process, many therapists recommend such self-help programs as Al-Anon, Children of Alcoholics, or Adult Children of Alcoholics.

Some recommend dietary changes (especially low-sugar diets), and such stress-reduction techniques as meditation, aerobics, and visualization or affirmation exercises.

Still, whatever form treatment takes, children of alcoholics need to develop a healthy sense of self-esteem—free of guilt, fear, and blame—to see themselves as okay even when those around them may not be.

It might seem like a cliché, but before any of us can ever really trust and love others, we really do have to learn to love and trust ourselves.

Pushing Past the Past

Perhaps the biggest trap that children of alcoholics can fall into is to see themselves—ourselves, since I'm one, too—as victims of horrible junk that's basically beyond our control and will somehow always keep us trapped.

That's not only self-defeating; it isn't even true.

Once you learn to see the past for what it is, past, and the present for what it is, a present, you're not going to find a good reason to be stopped by anything at all—especially mom or dad's problem or our memories of it.

Each of us may have had to grow up playing our parents' games, questioning our value, living in the shadow of alcoholism or chemical dependency.

But that doesn't mean we're stuck there. And even if we did learn to pretend that things were fine when they weren't, it's okay to stop pretending now.

How? By telling the truth about who we are and where we've been, and accepting and caring for ourselves—starting now, if you haven't started already.

There never has been—and never will be—a better time to put the past in its place. So why wait?

Getting Help

If you're worried about your drinking and you haven't been able to cut back or control it on your own, help is nearby.

Check the phone book for an alcohol information center or treatment program. The people there can tell you where and how to get help. It's never too early—or too late—to start.

If you can't find an alcohol information center in your area, phone or write either (or both) of the following:

- The National Council on Alcoholism and Drug Dependence, 12 West 21st Street, New York, NY 10010; (800) 622-2255.

- Alcoholics Anonymous, P.O. Box 459, Grand Central Station, New York, NY 10163

Just do it—and do it now. There'll never be a better time to get your life back on track.

Here's looking at you, kid—and at the person you can still become.

—by Lisa Turney

Chapter 42

Coping With An Alcoholic Parent

Anthony is already in bed when he hears the front door slam. He covers his head with his pillow to drown out the predictable sounds of his parents arguing. Anthony is all too aware that his father has been drinking again and his mother is angry.

Many teens like Anthony live with a parent who is an alcoholic, a person physically and emotionally addicted to alcohol. Alcoholism has been around for centuries, yet no one has discovered an easy way to prevent or stop it. Alcoholism continues to cause anguish not only for the person who drinks, but for everyone who is involved with that person.

According to the National Council on Alcoholism and Drug Dependence (NCADD), there are nearly 14 million Americans who are considered problem drinkers (including 8 million who have alcoholism) and 76 million people who are exposed to alcoholism in family settings. Although these rates show a huge number of problem drinkers, they also show that people who live with alcoholic family members are not alone.

About This Chapter: "Coping with an Alcoholic Parent," March 2007, reprinted with permission from www.kidshealth.org. Copyright © 2007 The Nemours Foundation. This information was provided by KidsHealth, one of the largest resources online for medically reviewed health information written for parents, kids, and teens. For more articles like this one, visit www.KidsHealth.org, or www.TeensHealth.org.

Why Does My Parent Drink?

Alcoholism is a disease. Like any disease, it needs to be treated. Without professional help, an alcoholic will probably continue to drink and may even become worse over time.

Just like any other disease, alcoholism is no one's fault. Some people who live with alcoholics blame themselves for their loved one's drinking. But the truth is, because of their disease, alcoholics would drink anyway. If your parent drinks, it won't change anything if you do better in school, help more

---

♣ It's A Fact!!
Does Your Mom Or Dad Drink Too Much?

Millions of youth like yourself worry about their parents drinking too much or using drugs. It's a big problem that happens in every kind of family, whether rich or poor, single parent, or traditional or blended family and families that attend places of worship.

When your parents have been drinking, do they show any of these symptoms?

• They embarrass you.

• They blame you for things you didn't do.

• They break promises.

• They drive under the influence.

• They behave in confusing and unpredictable ways.

Your parent could be misusing or be addicted to alcohol or drugs. Addiction to alcohol or drugs is a disease. People with this disease often do things that are confusing and hurtful. They need help to stop the alcohol or drug use. Sometimes that help is through an alcohol or drug abuse program; sometimes it is through Alcoholics Anonymous or other self-help groups, which often meet in churches and synagogues. These groups have helped millions of moms and dads recover, regain their health, and begin to heal their families. Caring adults are available to help your mom or dad get the treatment and recovery support they need.

Source: Excerpted from "It Feels So Bad—It Doesn't Have To," Substance Abuse and Mental Health Services Administration (SAMHSA), undated.

around the house, or do any of the other things you may believe your parent wants you to do.

Other people may tell themselves that their parents drink because of some other problem, such as having a rough time at work or being out of work altogether. Parents may be having marital problems, financial problems, or someone may be sick. But even if an alcoholic parent has other problems, nothing you can do will make things better. The person with the drinking problem has to take charge of it. No one else can help an alcoholic get well.

Why Won't My Parent Stop Drinking?

Denial can play a big role in an alcoholic's life. A person in denial is one who refuses to believe the truth about a situation. A problem drinker may blame another person for the drinking because it is easier than taking responsibility for it. Some alcoholic parents make their kids feel bad by saying things like, "You're driving me crazy!" or "I can't take this anymore."

An alcoholic parent may become enraged at the slightest suggestion that drinking is a problem. Those who acknowledge their drinking may show their denial by saying, "I can stop anytime I want to," "Everyone drinks to unwind sometimes," or "My drinking is not a problem."

Why Do I Feel So Bad?

If you're like most teens, your life is probably filled with emotional ups and downs, regardless of what's happening at home. Add a parent with a drinking problem to this tumultuous time and a person's bound to feel overwhelmed. Teens with alcoholic parents might feel anger, sadness, embarrassment, loneliness, helplessness, and a lack of self-esteem.

These emotions can be triggered by the added burdens of living with an alcoholic parent. For example, many alcoholics behave unpredictably, and kids who grow up around them may spend a lot of energy trying to feel out a parent's mood or guess what he or she wants. One day you might walk on eggshells to avoid an outburst because the dishes aren't done or the lawn isn't mowed; the next day, you may find yourself comforting a parent who promises that things will be better.

✔ Quick Tip
Dos And Don'ts For Children Of Alcoholics

Do talk about how you feel. You can talk with the safe people in your life—maybe a close friend, relative, school counselor, teacher, minister, or others. Sharing your feelings is not being mean to your family. Talking to someone about your feelings can help you feel less alone.

Do try to get involved in doing enjoyable things at school or near where you live—the school band, softball, Boy or Girl Scouts, or others. Doing these types of activities can help you forget about the problems at home, and you can learn new things about yourself and about how other people live their lives.

Do remember that feeling sad, afraid and alone is a normal way to feel when you live with alcoholic or drug-using parents. It's confusing to hate the disease of addiction at the same time that you love your parent. All people have confusing feelings, like having two different feelings at the same time. This is the way many kids feel about alcoholic or drug abusing parents.

Do remember to have fun. Sometimes children with addiction in their families worry so much that they forget how to be "just a kid." If things are bad at home, you might not have anyone who will help you have fun, but don't let that stop you. Find a way to let yourself have fun.

Don't ride in a car when the driver has been drinking if you can avoid it. It is not safe. Walk or try to get a ride with an adult friend who has not been drinking. If your parents are going out to drink somewhere, try not to go with them. If you must get in a car with a drinking driver, sit in the back seat in the middle. Lock your door. Put on your safety belt. Try to stay calm.

Don't think that because your parent has the disease of addiction that you will too. Most children of alcoholics do not become alcoholic themselves. While alcoholism does run in families, you can't get the disease if you don't drink or use drugs.

Don't pour out or try to water down your parent's alcohol. The plain fact is that it won't work. You have no control over the drinking. You didn't make the problem start, and you can't make it stop. It is up to your parent to get treatment and to recover. What your parent does is not your fault or your responsibility.

Source: From "Children of Alcoholics: A Kit For Educators," © 2001 National Association for Children of Alcoholics (www.nacoa.net). Reprinted with permission. To view the complete text of this booklet including references, visit http://www.nacoa.net/pdfs/EDkit_web_06.pdf. Despite the older date of this document, the suggestions offered are still pertinent.

There may be problems paying the bills, having your mom or dad show up for important events, and you may even have to take care of younger siblings, too. The pressure to manage these situations in addition to your own life—and maybe take care of younger siblings, too—can leave you exhausted and drained.

Although alcoholism causes similar patterns of damage to many families, each situation is unique. Some parents with alcohol problems might abuse their children emotionally or physically. Others neglect their kids by not providing sufficient care and guidance. Parents with alcohol problems may also use other drugs. Your family may have money troubles.

Although each family is different, teens with alcoholic parents almost always report feeling alone, unloved, depressed, or burdened by the secret life they lead at home. Because it's not possible to control the behavior of an alcoholic, what can a person do to feel better?

What Can I Do?

Teenage children of alcoholics are at a higher risk of becoming alcoholics themselves. Acknowledging the problem and reaching out for support can help ensure that your future does not repeat your parent's past.

Acknowledge the problem. An parent who is a problem drinker is never your fault. Many kids of alcoholics try to hide the problem or find themselves telling lies to cover up for a parent's drinking. Admitting that your parent has a problem—even if he or she won't—is the first step in taking control.

Being aware of how your parent's drinking affects you can help put things in perspective. For example, some teens who live with alcoholic adults become afraid to speak out or show any normal anger or emotion because they worry it may trigger a parent's drinking binge.

Clearly, hiding your feelings can create its own set of problems. Acknowledging feelings of anger or resentment—even if it's just to yourself or a close friend—can help protect against this. Recognizing the emotions that go with the problem also can help you from burying your feelings and pretending that everything's OK.

Likewise, realizing that you are not the cause of a parent's drinking problem can help you feel better about yourself.

Find support. It's good to share your feelings with a friend, but it's equally important to talk to an adult you trust. A school counselor, favorite teacher, or coach may be able to help. Some teens turn to their school D.A.R.E. (Drug and Alcohol Resistance Education) officer, whereas others find a sympathetic uncle or aunt.

Because alcoholism is such a widespread problem, several organizations offer support groups and meetings for people living with alcoholics. Al-Anon, an organization designed to help the families and friends of alcoholics, has a group called Alateen that is specifically geared to young people living with adults who have drinking problems. Alateen is not only for children of alcoholics, it can also help teens whose parents may already be in recovery. The group Alcoholics Anonymous (AA) also offers a variety of programs and resources for people living with alcoholics.

> ✔ Quick Tip
> **If It Is Your Friend's Mom Or Dad Who Drinks Too Much**
>
> Don't walk away, and don't pretend you don't see it.
>
> Here are some things that you can say that might help your friend.
>
> - It's not your fault that your parent drinks or uses drugs.
> - You're not alone—lots of kids come from families where this is a problem.
> - There are people who can help.
>
> Here are some things that you can do that might help your friend.
>
> - Tell your pastor or youth minister that you are worried about your friend.
> - Be a good friend—include your friend in your activities and your family's fun.
> - Encourage your friend to talk to a trusting adult.
>
> Source: Excerpted from "It Feels So Bad—It Doesn't Have To," Substance Abuse and Mental Health Services Administration (SAMHSA), undated.

You're not betraying your parent by seeking help. Keeping "the secret" is part of the disease of alcoholism—and it allows the problems to get worse. As with any disease, it's still possible to love a parent with alcoholism while recognizing the problems that he or she has. And it's not disloyal to seek help in dealing with the problems your parent's drinking create for you. In fact, taking care of yourself is what your dad or mom would want you to do if he or she could think about it clearly!

Find a safe environment. If you find yourself avoiding your house as much as possible, or if you're thinking about running away, consider whether you feel in danger at home. If you feel that the situation at home is becoming dangerous, you can call the National Domestic Violence Hotline at (800) 799-SAFE. And never hesitate to dial 911 if you think you or another family member is in immediate danger.

☞ Remember!!

Because alcoholism is a disease and not a behavior, chances are that you won't be able to change your parent's actions. But you can show your love and support—and, above all, take care of yourself.

Source: Nemours Foundation, 2007.

Chapter 43

Breaking The Cycle Of Alcohol Addiction

Children of alcoholics (COAs) are at increased risk for a wide range of behavioral and emotional problems, including addiction to alcohol and other drugs (AODs), depression, anxiety, school failure, and delinquency. Prevention and intervention efforts attempt to reduce this risk by modifying risk-associated factors. In general, prevention programs target children because of the behavior of an adult caregiver, rather than because of the child's own behavior. Intervention programs, however, usually target children who have begun to exhibit symptoms themselves, such as depression, poor academic performance, or problems getting along with their peers.

Several types of programs have been developed to assist COAs. Although a program may focus primarily on either prevention or intervention, most programs include elements of both. Therefore, this chapter discusses both types of programs somewhat interchangeably. In addition, the discussion primarily focuses on programs provided in group settings.

About This Chapter: This chapter includes excerpts from "Breaking The Cycle Of Addiction: Prevention And Intervention With Children Of Alcoholics," by Ann W. Price, M.A. and James G. Emshoff, Ph.D. *Alcohol Health and Research World*, National Institute on Alcohol Abuse and Alcoholism (NIAAA), Vol. 21, No. 3, 1997. The complete text of this article, including references, is available online at http://pubs.niaaa.nih.gov/publications/arh21-3/241.pdf. The information in this chapter was reviewed for currency by David A. Cooke, M.D., in December 2008.

> **☞ Remember!!**
> Children of alcoholics (COAs) are at increased risk for behavioral
> and emotional problems, including alcoholism. Research has helped guide
> the design of prevention and intervention programs aimed at reducing
> this risk.

Prevention Models

Primary prevention focuses on children who have not exhibited specific problems but who may be at risk because of genetic or environmental factors or both. Secondary prevention (that is, intervention) is targeted toward children who already exhibit behaviors predictive of later AOD use. Finally, the goal of tertiary prevention (which is analogous to treatment) is to help children who are already involved with AODs and to prevent further deterioration of their behavior.

Some research (Albee, GA. A manifesto for a fourth mental revolution? A review of the Report of the President's Commission on Mental Health. *Contemporary Psychology* 23:549-551, 1978) suggests that the risk for behavioral problems is increased by exposure to stress and reduced by social support, social competency (that is, social skills), and self-esteem. Therefore, the goals of primary prevention with COAs should include stress reduction and the development of self-esteem, social competence, and a strong social support system.

Other primary prevention models take a different approach. For example, the "distribution of consumption" model proposes to reduce the general public's consumption of alcohol by limiting its availability. This theoretically would reduce the number of problem drinkers and consequently the number of children exposed to alcohol problems in the family. This strategy involves raising the drinking age, limiting "happy hours," and increasing the price of alcoholic beverages or limiting the hours of their sale.

This approach will not be discussed here, however, because it does not specifically target COAs.

Another model, called the "sociocultural model," focuses on education and on enhancing children's competencies through information, values clarification (that is, examining values regarding alcohol), and skill-building techniques. The goal of this approach is to teach children to moderate their drinking and avoid later alcohol problems. Sociocultural programs can be implemented throughout the community or may be targeted via schools, recreational activities, or physicians' offices.

Screening And Identification

Many COAs never receive intervention services. COAs are usually identified incidentally when the child's parent enters alcoholism treatment. This type of identification is ineffective in reaching the majority of COAs, because most alcoholics never receive treatment. In addition, few children seek help voluntarily, because family denial puts pressure on the child to keep the family's secret.

Identification of COAs, therefore, requires a process of active screening. To this end, Dies and Burghardt (Group interventions for children of alcoholics: Prevention and treatment in the schools. *Journal of Adolescent Group Therapy* 1(3):219-234, 1991) describe certain behavior patterns that suggest a child may have an alcoholic parent. Some of these behaviors may reflect lack of parental supervision, such as frequent tardiness or absence from school or carelessness in dress or personal hygiene. Other

♣ **It's A Fact!!**

Despite their risk status, most COAs are remarkably well adjusted. Nevertheless, many children exhibit emotional and behavioral problems as a result of parental drinking. Improved research methods can guide intervention to prevent adverse outcomes from developing.

possible indicators of COA status include emotional instability, immaturity, conflict with peers, isolation from other children, academic problems, or physical complaints (for example, headaches and stomach aches). Many people who work with children are not trained to recognize these subtle signs; in addition, these signs are not specific to COAs. Therefore, researchers have

developed questionnaires to identify COAs who do not display obvious behavior problems.

One commonly used screening instrument is the CAGE, a set of four
questions regarding the respondent's concern over his or her own drinking
behavior. The Family CAGE is slightly reworded to reflect a respondent's
concern for the drinking habits of a relative. This questionnaire is intended
to screen for—not diagnose—family alcoholism; a positive finding on the
Family CAGE should be followed by a complete diagnostic assessment.

Another useful questionnaire is the Children of Alcoholics Screening Test
(CAST), designed to identify both young and adult children of alcoholics.
The 30-item instrument probes the respondent's attitudes, feelings, perceptions, and experiences related to the
drinking behavior of the respondent's parents. A shorter version of
CAST has also been developed.
Because of time constraints and the
fact that many school-based programs are run by teachers rather
than psychologists, such measures
are not routinely used to identify
COAs in the school environment.

Prevention Groups

Most programs for COAs are delivered in group settings. Group programs reduce COAs' feelings of
isolation, shame, and guilt while capitalizing on the importance to adolescents of peer influence and mutual
support. Groups may be structured
and closed-ended, with a specific beginning and end-point, or open-
ended, with participants joining and
leaving the group as they feel the need.

> ### ♣ It's A Fact!!
> ### The Family Cage:
> ### An Alcoholism Screening
> ### Test
>
> The CAGE is perhaps the most
> widely used screening test for alcohol-
> ism. This tool has been adapted to re-
> flect concern for a parent's drinking
> through the following four questions.
>
> 1. Do you think your parent needs
>   to cut (C) down on his/her
>   drinking?
>
> 2. Does your parent get annoyed
>   (A) comments about his/her
>   drinking?
>
> 3. Does your parent ever feel guilty
>   (G) about his/her drinking?
>
> 4. Does your parent ever take a
>   drink early in the morning as an
>   eye (E) opener?

Groups may be directed at the general population of COAs, as in broad-based community prevention programs, or targeted at specific high-risk groups, such as abused or neglected children as well as youth with academic problems or gang affiliations. These groups are readily identified and contain a large percentage of COAs. Prevention and intervention services can be offered to high-risk COAs as part of comprehensive social service programs aimed at those populations.

Alateen: Alateen is an example of a community based self-help program for COAs based on the 12-Step approach of Alcoholics Anonymous. Alateen generally meets in public settings, such as churches or community centers. Little data exist on the effectiveness of Alateen. In one study, COAs participating in Alateen had more positive scores than nonparticipating COAs on a scale measuring mood and self-esteem, factors affecting risk for behavioral problems, including alcohol misuse. Conversely, in a study of four- to 16-year-old sons of alcoholics, one researcher found that group counseling had more positive effects than did Alateen in improving self-worth (Peitler, EJ. A comparison of the effectiveness of group counseling and Alateen on the psychological adjustment of two groups of adolescent sons of alcoholic fathers. *Dissertation Abstracts International* 41:152B, 1980). Unfortunately, not enough empirical evidence exists to draw any firm conclusions about the effectiveness of Alateen.

School-Based Groups: Children are available at schools for long periods of time and in large numbers; therefore, educational institutions are logical settings for intervention efforts. Behavior problems potentially indicating parental alcoholism can be most readily recognized in school. An added benefit is that COA programs within schools have ready access to needed information and services. Finally, children and adolescents may find it embarrassing to attend programs at an outside agency or treatment center, particularly in settings that may have a negative stigma attached (for example, mental health centers).

Program Content

Although there are several types of intervention programs, some strategies are common to most programs. Among these strategies are training in social competency and coping skills, as well as providing information, social support, and alternatives to AOD use. These strategies have been developed for prevention efforts with diverse populations, but are applied (and sometimes adapted or customized) to groups of COAs.

The content of COA prevention and intervention programs is often based on social cognitive theory. The goals of such programs are to reduce children's stress, increase their social support system, provide specific competencies and skills, and provide opportunities for increased self-esteem. Social cognitive theory emphasizes techniques such as role-playing, modeling, practice of resistance skills, and feedback. Role-playing allows the child to rehearse common situations such as riding in the car with a drunk parent. Through modeling, participants learn appropriate behavior (for example, effective communication skills) by observing group leaders and peers. Resistance skills help children cope with peer pressure to drink. Both the group leader and participants provide the child with positive feedback to reinforce and encourage newly acquired skills. These techniques have contributed to significant reductions in the use of cigarettes, alcohol, and marijuana in general prevention programs that target wider groups rather than COAs specifically. More research is needed to test these techniques with COAs.

♣ It's A Fact!!
The influence of the child's developmental stage must be considered during program design. For example, elementary school-aged children do not always have realistic perceptions of relationships and causal links and may believe that they are the cause of their parents' drinking problem.

During the middle school years, COAs, as well as other children, often make decisions about using AODs themselves. In addition, the emergence of emotional or mental health problems is not unusual for many adolescents, including COAs. Therefore, prevention efforts should focus on the preteen years.

Many COAs who appear to be coping well are actually in a self-protective state of denial. Group facilitators should exercise patience and sensitivity as children adjust to their changing awareness about their parents' drinking.

Group leaders should also recognize that COAs may become overly dependent on them and should be sensitive to the feelings of abandonment that children may experience when the group terminates.

Information And Education: Most programs provide information about alcohol and alcoholism to help correct false expectancies. For example, COAs often overestimate the positive effects of alcohol consumption on cognitive and social performance, thereby increasing their risk for excessive drinking.

Most programs promote the concept of alcoholism as a disease to help the child put the behavior of the alcoholic parent in perspective. For example, understanding the biological basis of alcoholism manifestations such as tolerance, blackouts, and withdrawal helps the child overcome misplaced self-blame and guilt about parental drinking. Finally, COAs must learn that they are at risk for a variety of psychosocial problems, especially alcoholism. Research shows that COAs who are aware of their risk status drink significantly less than COAs who are unaware of their risk status.

Competencies And Coping Skills: Competencies are skills that help children cope with stress, thereby reducing their risk for alcoholism and other psychosocial problems. Most programs teach specific emotion-focused and problem-focused coping skills. Emotion-focused coping is a process by which the child seeks social support or uses strategies such as distancing or reframing the negative aspects of the situation to emphasize the positive aspects. For example, the child's inability to control parental drinking may be offset by the knowledge that sources of help are available.

Problem-focused coping emphasizes the problems of living in an alcoholic home, such as having to explain unusual parental behavior to friends. In addition, this approach attempts to enhance decision making, problem-solving, and communication skills, as well as the ability to resist peer pressure to drink. Emotion-focused and problem-focused skills are not mutually exclusive, and children who learn both skills are better equipped to manage their lives.

Personal-Social Competencies: Personal-social competencies can improve COA functioning despite exposure to stress. Such competencies include the ability to establish and maintain intimate relationships, express feelings, and solve problems. These skills can be enhanced by buttressing the COAs self-esteem and self-efficacy (that is, the belief that one can perform a particular task).

Social support arises naturally out of participation in group treatment. In the group setting, children often learn for the first time that other children have problems similar to theirs. Many children benefit from sharing their experiences and emotions in a safe environment with other children. Through mutual exchange, children learn survival skills from the experiences of their peers, gain practice in expressing feelings, and build their social support networks.

♣ It's A Fact!!

Many COAs attempt to achieve perfection in everything they do as a means of acquiring self-esteem. This sets the stage for inevitable failure. Therefore, interventions often emphasize alternative ways to acquire self-esteem and self-efficacy.

Alternative Activities: Alternative activities provide opportunities for COAs to participate in activities that exclude alcohol, tobacco, and other drugs. Healthy alternative activities (for example, sports, peer leadership training institutes, and programs such as Outward Bound) may help children build a sense of self-efficacy; increase self-esteem; provide a positive peer group; and increase life skills, such as problem-solving and communication. Programs may focus exclusively on alternative activities but preferably are part of a comprehensive prevention program.

Part Seven

If You Need More Information

Chapter 44

Additional Reading About Alcohol Use And Abuse

Books

Big Book Unplugged:
A Young Person's Guide to Alcoholics Anonymous
By John R.
Published by Hazelden, 2003

The Big Deal About Alcohol:
What Teens Need To Know About Drinking
By Marilyn McClellan
Published by Enslow Publishers, 2004

Drowning In A Bottle:
Teens And Alcohol Abuse
By Gail Stewart
Published by Compass Point Books, 2009

About This Chapter: The books, webpages, magazines, and newsletters in this chapter were selected from a wide variety of sources deemed accurate. Inclusion does not constitute endorsement. To make topics readily apparent, these resources are listed alphabetically by title within each category.

From Binge To Blackout:
A Mother And Son Struggle With Teen Drinking
By Chris Volkmann and Toren Volkmann
Published by Penguin Group, 2006

I've Got This Friend Who: Advice For Teens And Their Friends
On Alcohol, Drugs, Eating Disorders, Risky Behavior And More
By KidsPeace
Published by Hazelden, 2007

Living With Alcoholism And Addiction
By Nicholas R. Lessa and Sara D. Gilbert
Published by Facts on File, 2009

On The Rocks: Teens And Alcohol
By David Aretha
Published by Childrens Press, 2007

When Someone You Love Abuses Alcohol or Drugs:
A Guide for Kids
By James J. Crist, Ph.D.
Published by Wellness Institute, 2003

Young, Sober and Free:
Teen-to-Teen Stories of Hope and Recovery
By Shelly Marshall
Published by Hazelden, 2003

Webpages, Magazines, And Newsletters

AA Grapevine Magazine
Alcoholics Anonymous
http://www.aagrapevine.org

Alcohol Abuse Health Center
WebMD
http://www.webmd.com/mental-health/alcohol-abuse/default.htm

Alcohol Alert Series
National Institute On Alcohol Abuse And Alcoholism
http://www.niaaa.nih.gov/Publications/AlcoholAlerts/default.htm

Alcohol Online Tests
Substance Abuse And Mental Health Services Administration
http://getfit.samhsa.gov/alcohol/tests/default.aspx?postion=2

Check Yourself
http://www.checkyourself.com

The Cool Spot
National Institute On Alcohol Abuse And Alcoholism
http://www.thecoolspot.gov

Do It Now Foundation
http://www.doitnow.org

Free Vibe
National Youth Anti-Drug Media Campaign
http://www.freevibe.com

Go Ask Alice
Columbia University
http://www.goaskalice.columbia.edu

National Alcohol And Drug Addiction Recovery Month
Substance Abuse and Mental Health Services Administration
http://www.recoverymonth.gov

National Clearing House For Alcohol And Drug Information
Substance Abuse and Mental Health Services Administration
http://ncadi.samhsa.gov

NIDA For Teens
National Institute On Drug Abuse (NIDA)
http://www.teens.drugabuse.gov

Overboard
PBS Online
http://www.thirteen.org/closetohome/overboard/menu.html

Stop Underage Drinking
A Portal of Federal Resources
http://www.stopalcoholabuse.gov

Too Smart To Start Youth Pages
Substance Abuse and Mental Health Services Administration
http://toosmarttostart.samhsa.gov/youth/youth.aspx

Chapter 45

Support Groups For Alcoholics And Children Of Alcoholics

Adult Children Of Alcoholics World Service Organization, Inc.

P.O. Box 3216
Torrance, CA 90510-3216
Phone: 310-534-1815 (message only)
Website: http://www.adultchildren.org
E-mail: info@adultchildren.org

About This Chapter: The list of organizations in this chapter was compiled from many sources deemed accurate. Inclusion does not constitute endorsement. There is no implication associated with omission. All contact information was verified in February 2009.

Al-Anon/Alateen Family Groups

Al-Anon Family Group Headquarters, Inc.
Al-Anon Family Group Headquarters (Canada) Inc.
1600 Corporate Landing Parkway
Virginia Beach, VA 23454-5617
Phone: 757-563-1600
Fax: 757-563-1655
Website: http://www.al-anon.alateen.org
E-mail: wso@al-anon.org

Alcoholics Anonymous

A.A. World Services, Inc.
P.O. Box 459
New York, NY 10163
Phone: 212-870-3400
Fax: 212-870-3003
Website: http://www.aa.org

Alcoholics For Christ

1316 North Campbell Road
Royal Oak, MI 48067
Toll-Free: 800-441-7877
Phone: 248-399-9955
Fax: 248-399-1099
Website: http://
www.alcoholicsforchrist.com
E-mail:al4christ333@sbcglobal.net

Alcoholics Victorious

4501 Troost Ave.
Kansas City, MO 64110-4127
Phone: 816-561-0567
Fax: 816-561-0572
Website: http://
www.alcoholicsvictorious.org

Calix Society

International Office
3881 Highland Avenue
Suite 201
White Bear Lake, MN 55110
Toll-Free: 800-398-0524
Phone: 651-773-3117
Website: http://www.calixsociety.org

Celebrate Recovery

Website: http://
www.celebraterecovery.com
Click on "Find a Group" to find a
location in your state.
E-mail:
info@celebraterecovery.com

Centre For Addiction And Mental Health

33 Russell Street
Toronto, ON M5S 2S1
Canada
Toll Free: 800-463-6273
Phone: 416-535-8501
Website: http://www.camh.net

Chemically Dependent Anonymous

General Service Office
P.O. Box 423
Severna Park, MD 21146
Toll-Free: 888-232-4673
Website: http://www.cdaweb.org

Children Of Alcoholics Foundation

164 West 74th Street
New York, NY 10023
Toll Free: 800-488-DRUG (3784)
Phone: 646-505-2060
Fax: 212-595-2553
Website: http://www.coaf.org
E-mail: coaf@phoenixhouse.org

Christian Harbor Family Alcoholism Recovery

P.O. Box 266
El Reno, OK 73036
Website: http://
www.christianharbor.com

DailyStrength

12121 Wilshire Boulevard
Suite 1100
Los Angeles, CA 90025
Website: http://dailystrength.org

Do It Now Foundation

P.O. Box 27568
Tempe, AZ 85285-7568
Phone: 480-736-0599
Fax: 480-736-0771
Website: http://www.doitnow.org
E-mail: email@doitnow.org

Double Trouble In Recovery, Inc.

P.O. Box 245055
Brooklyn, NY 11224
Phone: 718-373-2684
Website: http://
www.doubletroubleinrecovery.org

Dual Recovery Anonymous

World Services Central Office
P.O. Box 8107
Prairie Village, KS 66208
Phone: 913-991-2703 (afternoons)
Website: http://draonline.org
E-mail: draws@draonline.org

Families Anonymous

P.O. Box 3475
Culver City, CA 90231-3475
Toll-Free: 800-736-9805
Fax: 310-815-9682
Website: http://
www.familiesanonymous.org
E-mail:
famanon@FamiliesAnonymous.org

Free N One Recovery

5838 South Overhill Drive
Suite 2
Los Angeles, CA 90043
Phone: 323-295-0009

Inspire

P.O. Box 1438
Princeton, NJ 08540
Toll-Free: 800-945-0381
Phone: 703-243-0303
Fax: 202-478-0377
Website: www.inspire.com
E-mail: team@inspire.com

Jewish Alcoholics, Chemically Dependent Persons, And Significant Others (JACS)

120 West 57th Street
New York, NY 10019
Phone: 212-397-4197
Fax: 212-399-3525
Website: http://www.jacsweb.org
E-mail: jacs@jacsweb.org

LifeRing Secular Recovery

LifeRing Service Center
1440 Broadway, Suite 312
Oakland CA 94612
Toll-Free: 800-811-4142
Phone: 510-763-0779
Fax 510-763-1513
Website: http://
www.unhooked.com
E-mail: service@lifering.org

Men For Sobriety

P.O. Box 618
Quakertown, PA 18951-0618
Phone: 215-536-8026
Fax: 215-538-9026
E-mail: NewLife@nni.com

Moderation Management Network, Inc.

22 West 27th Street, 5th Floor
New York, NY 10001
Website: http://moderation.org

National Association For Children Of Alcoholics

11426 Rockville Pike, Suite 301
Rockville, MD 20852
Toll-Free: 888-55-4COAS (2627)
Phone: 301-468-0985
Fax: 301-468-0987
Website: http://
www.childrenofalcoholics.org
E-mail: nacoa@nacoa.org

National Center On Addiction And Substance Abuse At Columbia University

633 Third Avenue, 19th Floor
New York, NY 10017-6706
Phone: 212-841-5200
Website: http://
www.casacolumbia.org

Overcomers In Christ

P.O. Box 34460
Omaha, NE 68134-0460
Website: http://
www.OvercomersInChrist.org
E-mail:
info@overcomersinchrist.org

Overcomers Outreach, Inc.

12828 Acheson Drive
Whittier, CA 90601
Toll-Free: 800-310-3001
Phone: 562-698-9000
Fax: 562-698-2211
Website: http://
www.overcomersoutreach.org
E-mail:
info@overcomersoutreach.org

Overcomer's Recovery Support Program

P.O. Box 29623
Shreveport, LA 71149-9623
Phone: 318-687-4777
Fax: 318-687-5777
Website: http://recoverysupport.org

Recoveries Anonymous

R.A. Universal Services
P.O. Box 1212
East Northport, NY 11731
Website: http://www.r-a.org
E-mail: raus@r-a.org

Recovery, Inc.

105 W. Adams, Suite 2940
Chicago, IL 60603
Toll-Free: 866-221-0302
Phone: 312-337-5661
Fax: 312-726-4446
Website: http://recovery-inc.org
E-mail: inquiries@recovery-inc.org

Secular Organizations For Sobriety (Save Ourselves)

4773 Hollywood Boulevard
Hollywood, CA 90027
Website: http://www.cfiwest.org/sos
E-mail: SOS@CFIWest.org

SMART Recovery Self-Help Network

7537 Mentor Avenue, Suite 306
Mentor, OH 44060
Toll-Free: 866-951-5357
Phone: 440-951-5357
Fax: 440-951-5358
Website: http://
www.smartrecovery.org
E-mail: info@smartrecovery.org

SoberCircle

Website: http://
www.sobercircle.com
E-mail:
webmaster@sobercircle.com

Substance Abuse Treatment Facility Locator

Substance Abuse And Mental
Health Services Administration
5600 Fishers Lane
Rockville, MD 20857
Website: http://
www.findtreatment.samhsa.gov

Teen-Anon

Streetcats Foundation for Youth
and National Children's Coalition
P.O. Box 72176
Oakland, CA 94612
Website: http://www.teen-anon.com
E-mail: teenanon@yahoo.com

Women For Sobriety, Inc.

P.O. Box 618
Quakertown, PA 18951-0618
Phone: 215-536-8026
Fax: 215-538-9026
Website: http://
www.womenforsobriety.org

Chapter 46

National Organizations Providing Information About Alcohol And Alcoholism

Federal Agencies

Agency For Healthcare Research And Quality

540 Gaither Road
Suite 2000
Rockville, MD 20850
Clearinghouse Toll-Free:
800-358-9295
Clearinghouse TTY: 888-586-6340
Phone: 301-427-1364
Website: http://www.ahrq.gov
E-mail: info@ahrq.gov

Bureau Of Alcohol, Tobacco, Firearms And Explosives

Office of Public and Governmental Affairs
99 New York Ave. N.E.
Washington, DC 20226
Toll-Free: 888-800-3855
Phone: 202-648-7777
Website: http://www.atf.treas.gov
E-mail: ATFMail@atf.gov

Centers For Disease Control And Prevention (CDC)

1600 Clifton Road
Atlanta, GA 30333
Toll-Free: 800-CDC-INFO
(800-232-4636)
Phone: 404-639-3311
Website: http://www.cdc.gov

Healthfinder®
U.S. Department of Health and
Human Services
P.O. Box 1133
Washington, DC 20013-1133
Website: http://
www.healthfinder.gov
E-mail: healthfinder@nhic.org

**National Center For Health
Statistics**
3311 Toledo Road
Hyattsville, MD 20782
Toll-Free: 866-441-NCHS
(441-6247)
Phone: 301-458-4000
Website: http://www.cdc.gov/nchs
E-mail: nchsquery@cdc.gov

**National Clearinghouse For
Alcohol And Drug
Information**
Toll-Free: 800-729-6686
Toll-Free TDD: 800-487-4889
Website: http://ncadi.samhsa.gov

**National Health Information
Center**
P.O. Box 1133
Washington, DC 20013
Toll-Free: 800-336-4797
Phone: 301-565-4167
Website: http://www.health.gov/nhic
E-mail: info@nhic.org

**National Highway Traffic
Safety Administration**
NHTSA Headquarters
1200 New Jersey Avenue, S.E.
West Building
Washington, DC 20590
Toll-Free: 888-327-4236
Toll-Free TTY: 800-424-9153
Website: http://www.nhtsa.gov

**National Institute Of Child
Health And Human
Development**
Bldg. 31, Room 2A32, MSC 2425
31 Center Drive
Bethesda, MD 20892-2425
Toll-Free: 800-370-2943
TTY: 888-320-6942
Website: http://www.nichd.nih.gov
E-mail: NICHDInformation
ResourceCenter@mail.nih.gov

**National Institute Of
Diabetes And Digestive And
Kidney Diseases**
National Institutes of Health
Building 31, Room 9A04
31 Center Drive, MSC 2560
Bethesda, MD 20892-2560
Information Clearinghouse
Toll-Free: 800-891-5390
NIDDK Programs: 301-496-3583
Website: http://www.niddk.nih.gov
E-mail:
dkwebmaster@extra.niddk.nih.gov

National Institute Of Neurological Disorders And Stroke

P.O. Box 5801
Bethesda, MD 20824
Toll-Free: 800-352-9424
Phone: 301-496-5751
TTY: 301-468-5981
Website: http://www.ninds.nih.gov
E-mail: braininfo@ninds.nih.gov

National Institute On Alcohol Abuse And Alcoholism

5635 Fishers Lane, MSC 9304
Bethesda, MD 20892-9304
Websites: http://
www.niaaa.nih.gov; http://
www.collegedrinkingprevention.gov
E-mail: niaaaweb-r@exchange.nih.gov

National Institute On Drug Abuse

6001 Executive Blvd., Room 5213
Bethesda, MD 20892-9561
Phone: 301-443-1124
Website: http://www.nida.nih.gov
E-mail: information@nida.nih.gov

National Institutes Of Health

9000 Rockville Pike
Bethesda, MD 20892
Phone: 301-496-4000
Website: http://www.nih.gov
E-mail: NIHinfo@OD.nih.gov

National Women's Health Information Center

8270 Willow Oaks Corporate Drive
Fairfax, VA 22031
Toll-Free: 800-994-9662
TTY: 888-220-5446
Website: http://www.4woman.gov

National Youth Anti-Drug Media Campaign

White House Office of National
Drug Control Policy
Drug Policy Information
Clearinghouse
P.O. Box 6000
Rockville, MD 20849-6000
Toll-Free: 800-666-3332
Fax: 301-519-6212
Website:
www.whitehousedrugpolicy.gov
E-mail: ondcp@ncjrs.org

Office Of Minority Health

U.S. Department of Health and
Human Services
The Tower Building
1101 Wootton Parkway, Suite 600
Rockville, MD 20852
Toll-Free: 800-444-6472
Phone: 240-453-2882
Fax: 240-453-2883
Website: http://www.omhrc.gov
E-mail: info@omhrc.gov

Office Of Safe And Drug-Free Schools

U.S. Department of Education
550 12th St. S.W., 10th Floor
At Potomac Center Plaza
Washington, DC 20202-6450
Toll-Free: 800-624-0100
(Publication Center)
Phone: 202-245-7896
Fax: 202-485-0013
Website: http://www.ed.gov/about/
offices/list/osdfs/index.html
E-mail: osdfs.safeschl@ed.gov

Substance Abuse And Mental Health Services Administration

P.O. Box 2345
Rockville, MD 20847
Toll-Free: 877-SAMHSA-7
(877-726-4727)
Fax: 240-221-4292
Website: http://www.samhsa.gov

U.S. Department Of Education

400 Maryland Avenue, S.W.
Washington, DC 20202
Toll-Free: 800-872-5327
Toll-Free TTY: 800-437-0833
Fax: 202-401-0689
Website: http://www.ed.gov

U.S. Food And Drug Administration

10903 New Hampshire Ave.
Silver Spring, MD 20903
Toll-Free: 888-463-6332
(888-INFO-FDA)
Website: http://www.fda.gov

U.S. National Library Of Medicine

8600 Rockville Pike
Bethesda, MD 20894
Toll-Free: 888-346-3656
Phone: 301-594-5983
Website: http://www.nlm.nih.gov
E-mail: custserv@nlm.nih.gov

Private, Civic, And Religious Organizations

Advertising Council

815 2nd Ave., 9th Floor
New York, NY 10017
Phone: 212-922-1500
Website: http://www.adcouncil.org

Alcoholics Anonymous (AA)

A.A. World Services, Inc.
P.O. Box 459
New York, NY 10163
Phone: 212-870-3400
Website: http://www.aa.org

American Council For Drug Education

164 West 74th Street
New York, NY 10023
Toll-Free: 800-488-3784
Website: http://www.acde.org
E-mail: acde@phoenixhouse.org

American Liver Foundation

75 Maiden Lane, Suite 603
New York, NY 10038
Toll-Free: 800-465-4837 (helpline)
Phone: 212-668-1000
Fax: 212-483-8179
Website: http://
www.liverfoundation.org
E-mail: info@liverfoundation.org

American Psychological Association

750 First Street, N.E.
Washington, DC 20002-4242
Toll-Free: 800-374-2721
Phone: 202-336-5500
TDD/TTY: 202-336-6123
Website: http://www.apa.org

American Public Health Association

800 I Street, N.W.
Washington, DC 20001-3710
Phone: 202-777-2742
Fax: 202-777-2534
Website: http://www.apha.org
E-mail: comments@apha.org

American Society Of Addiction Medicine

4601 North Park Avenue
Arcade Suite 101
Chevy Chase, MD 20815
Phone: 301-656-3920
Fax: 301-656-3815
Website: http://www.asam.org
E-mail: email@asam.org

Association For Medical Education And Research In Substance Abuse

125 Whipple Street, Third Floor
Suite 300
Providence, RI 02908
Phone: 401-243-8460
Fax: 877-418-8769
Website: http://www.amersa.org

Canadian Centre On Substance Abuse

75 Albert Street, Suite 300
Ottawa, ON K1P 5E7
Canada
Phone: 613-235-4048
Fax: 613-235-8101
Website: http://www.ccsa.ca
E-mail: info@ccsa.ca

Caron Foundation

P.O. Box 150
Wernersville, PA 19565
Toll-Free: 800-678-2332
Website: http://www.caron.org
E-mail: info@caron.org

Center For Substance Abuse Research

University of Maryland
4321 Hartwick Road, Suite 501
College Park, MD 20740
Phone: 301-405-9770
Fax: 301-403-8342
Website: http://www.cesar.umd.edu

Center Of Alcohol Studies

Rutgers, The State University of
New Jersey
607 Allison Road
Piscataway, NJ 08854-8001
Phone: 732-445-2190
Fax: 732-445-3500
Website: http://
www.alcoholstudies.rutgers.edu
E-mail: chrouse@rci.rutgers.edu

The Century Council

2345 Crystal Drive, Suite 910
Arlington, VA 22202
Phone: 202-637-0077
Website: http://
www.centurycouncil.org

Do It Now Foundation

P.O. Box 27568
Tempe, AZ 85285-7568
Phone: 480-736-0599
Fax: 480-736-0771
Website: http://www.doitnow.org/
pages/nowhome2.html
E-mail: e-mail@doitnow

Dual Recovery Anonymous

World Services Central Office
P.O. Box 8107
Prairie Village, KS 66208
Phone: 913-991-2703 (afternoons)
Website: http://www.draonline.org
E-mail: draws@draonline.org

Ensuring Solutions To Alcohol Problems

George Washington University
2021 K Street N.W., Suite 800
Washington, DC 20006
Phone: 202-296-6922
Fax: 202-296-0025
Website: http://
www.ensuringsolutions.org
E-mail: info@ensuringsolutions.org

FACE® Truth And Clarity On Alcohol

105 West Fourth Street
Clare, MI 48617
Toll-Free: 888-822-3223
Fax: 989-386-3532
Website: http://www.faceproject.org
E-mail: face@faceproject.org

Betty Ford Center

39000 Bob Hope Drive
Rancho Mirage, CA 92270
Toll-Free: 800-434-7365
Phone: 760-773-4100
Fax: 760-773-4126
Website: http://
www.bettyfordcenter.org

Hazelden Foundation
CO3, P.O. Box 11
Center City, MN 55012-0011
Toll-Free: 800-257-7810
Phone: 651-213-4200
Website: www.hazelden.org
E-mail: info@hazelden.org

Institute Of Alcohol Studies
Alliance House
12 Caxton Street
London SW1H 0QS
Phone: +44 (0) 207-222-4001
Fax: +44 (0) 207-799-2510
Website: http://www.ias.org.uk
E-mail: info@ias.org.uk

Jewish Alcoholics, Chemically Dependent Persons, And Significant Others
120 West 57th St.
New York, NY 10019
Phone: 212-397-4197
Fax: 212-399-3525
Website: http://www.jacsweb.org
E-mail: jacs@jacsweb.org

Johnson Institute
Executive Office
613 Second St., N.E.
Washington, DC 20002
Website: http://www.johnsoninstitute.org

Join Together
715 Albany Street
580-3rd Floor
Boston, MA 02118
Phone: 617-437-1500
Fax: 617-437-9394
Website: http://www.jointogether.org
E-mail: info@jointogether.org

Juvenile Justice Clearinghouse
National Criminal Justice
Reference Service
P.O. Box 6000
Rockville, MD 20849-6000
Toll-Free: 800-638-8736
Toll-Free TTY: 877–712–9279
TTY: 301–947–8374
Fax: 410–792–4358 (to order publications by title or number)
Fax: 301-519-5212 (for other assistance)
Website: http://www.ojjdp.ncjrs.org
E-mail: puborder@ncjrs.org (to order publications by title or number)
E-mail: askncjrs@ncjrs.org (for other assistance)

Kaiser Family Foundation
2400 Sand Hill Road
Menlo Park, CA 94025
Phone: 650-854-9400
Fax: 650-854-4800
Website: http://www.kff.org

Leadership To Keep Children Alcohol-Free

c/o The CDM Group, Inc.
7500 Old Georgetown Road
Suite 900
Bethesda, MD 20814
Phone: 301-654-6740
Fax: 301-656-4012
Website: http://
www.alcoholfreechildren.org
E-mail:
leadership@alcoholfreechildren.org

Marin Institute

24 Belvedere Street
San Rafael, CA 94901
Phone: 415-456-5692
Website: http://
www.marininstitute.org
E-mail: info@marininstitute.org

Mothers Against Drunk Driving (MADD)

MADD National Office
511 E. John Carpenter Freeway
Suite 700
Irving, TX 75062
Toll-Free: 800-438-6233
(800-GET-MADD)
Toll-Free: 877-623-3435 (Victim Services)
Phone: 214-744-6233
Fax: 972-869-2206; 972-869-2207
Website: http://www.madd.org

National Association Of Addiction Treatment Providers

313 W. Liberty Street
Suite 129
Lancaster, PA 17603-2748
Phone: 717-392-8480
Fax: 717-392-8481
Website: http://www.naatp.org
E-mail: rhunsicker@naatp.org

National Association Of Alcoholism And Drug Abuse Counselors

1001 N. Fairfax St.
Suite 201
Alexandria, VA 22314
Toll-Free: 800-548-0497
Phone 703-741-7686
Fax: 703-741-7698
Website: http://www.naadac.org
E-mail: naadac@naadac.org

National Association Of State Alcohol And Drug Abuse Directors

1025 Connecticut Ave. N.W.
Suite 605
Washington, DC 20036
Phone: 202-293-0090
Fax: 202-293-1250
Website: http://www.nasadad.org
E-mail: dcoffice@nasadad.org

National Association On Alcohol, Drugs And Disability, Inc.
2165 Bunker Hill Drive
San Mateo, CA 94402-3801
Website: http://www.naadd.org

National Center On Addiction And Substance Abuse At Columbia University
633 Third Avenue, 19th Floor
New York, NY 10017-6706
Phone: 212-841-5200
Website: http://www.casacolumbia.org

National Council On Alcoholism And Drug Dependence
244 East 58th Street. 4th Floor
New York, NY 10022
Toll-Free: 800-622-2255
Phone: 212-269-7797
Fax: 212-269-7510
Website: http://www.ncadd.org
E-mail: national@ncadd.org

National Safety Council
1121 Spring Lake Drive
Itasca, IL 60143-3201
Toll-Free: 800-621-7615
Phone: 630-285-1121
Fax: 630-285-1315
Website: http://www.nsc.org
E-mail: customerservice@nsc.org

Partnership For A Drug-Free America
405 Lexington Avenue
Suite 1601
New York, NY 10174
Phone: 212-922-1560
Fax: 212-922-1570
Website: http://www.drugfree.org

Phoenix House
164 West 74th Street
Toll-Free: 800-378-4435
(800-DRUG-HELP)
New York, NY 10023
Phone: 212-595-5810
Website: http://
www.phoenixhouse.org

Red Ribbon Works
200 Mills Avenue
P.O. Box 10203
Greenville, SC 29603
Phone: 800-732-4099
Fax: 864-467-4102
Website: http://
www.redribbonworks.org

RID (Remove Intoxicated Drivers) USA, Inc.
P.O. Box 520
Schenectady, NY 12301
Phone: 518-393-4357
Fax: 518-370-4917
Website: http://www.rid-usa.org
E-mail: dwi@rid-usa.org

Secular Organizations For Sobriety (SOS)
4773 Hollywood Boulevard
Hollywood, CA 90027
Website: http://www.sossobriety.org

Students Against Destructive Decisions (SADD)
255 Main Street
Marlborough, MA 01752
Toll-Free: 877-723-3462
(877-SADD-INC)
Fax: 508-481-5759
Website: http://www.sadd.org
E-mail: info@sadd.org

Women For Sobriety, Inc.
P.O. Box 618
Quakertown, PA 18951-0618
Phone: 215-536-8026
Fax: 215-538-9026
Website: http://
www.womenforsobriety.org
E-mail: NewLife@nni.com

Resources For Children Of Alcoholics

Adult Children Of Alcoholics World Service Organization, Inc.
P.O. Box 3216
Torrance, CA 90510-3216
Website: http://www.adultchildren.org
E-mail: info@adultchildren.org

Al-Anon/Alateen Family Groups
Al-Anon Family Group
Headquarters, Inc.
Al-Anon Family Group
Headquarters (Canada) Inc.
1600 Corporate Landing Parkway
Virginia Beach, VA 23454-5617
Phone: 757-563-1600
Fax: 757-563-1655
Website: http://www.al-anon
.alateen.org
E-mail: wso@al-anon.org

Intervention Resource Center, Inc.
1028 Barret Avenue
Louisville, KY 40204
Toll-Free: 888-421-4321
Fax: 502-451-1337
Website: http://
www.interventioninfo.org
E-mail: help@interventioninfo.org

National Association For Children Of Alcoholics
11426 Rockville Pike
Suite 301
Rockville, MD 20852
Toll-Free: 888-554-2627
Phone: 301-468-0985
Fax: 301-468-0987
Websites: http://www.nacoa.net;
http://www.childrenofalcoholics.org
E-mail: nacoa@nacoa.org

Resources About Alcohol-Related Birth Defects

The Arc Of The United States

Main Office
1010 Wayne Avenue
Suite 650
Silver Spring, MD 20910
Toll-Free: 800-433-5255
Phone: 301-565-3842
Fax: 301-565-3843; 301-565-5342
Website: http://www.thearc.org
E-mail: info@thearc.org

Family Empowerment Network

Great Lakes FASD Regional
Training Center
University of Wisconsin School of
Medicine and Public Health
Department of Family Medicine
777 S. Mills Street
Madison, WI 53715
Toll-Free: 800752-3157
Phone: 608-261-1418
Fax: 608-263-5813
Website: http://
pregnancyandalcohol.org
E-mail: FASD.trainingcenter
@fammed.wisc.edu

March Of Dimes

1275 Mamaroneck Avenue
White Plains, NY 10605
National Office Phone:
914-997-4488
Website: http://
www.marchofdimes.com

National Organization On Fetal Alcohol Syndrome (NOFAS)

900 17th Street, N.W.
Suite 910
Washington, DC 20006
Toll-Free: 800-666-6327
(800-66NOFAS)
Phone: 202-785-4585
Fax: 202-466-6456
Website: http://www.nofas.org

National Center On Birth Defects And Development

Fetal Alcohol Syndrome Prevention
Section
Centers For Disease Control And
Prevention
4770 Buford Highway, N.E.
MSF-49
Atlanta, GA 30341-3724
Fax: 770-488-7361
Website: http://www.cdc.gov/
ncbddd

Chapter 47

State Resources For Help With Alcohol-Related Concerns

Alabama

Substance Abuse Services Division
Department of Mental Health/
Retardation
P.O. Box 301410
100 North Union Street
Montgomery, AL 36130-1410
Phone: 334-242-3454
Fax: 334-242-0725
Website: http://www.mh.alabama.gov
E-mail:
DMHMR@MH.Alabama.gov

About This Chapter: The information in this chapter was compiled from "Substance Abuse Treatment Facility Locator," Substance Abuse and Mental Health Services Administration (SAMHSA), U.S. Department of Health and Human Services. Inclusion does not constitute endorsement. All contact information was verified in February 2009.

Alaska

Division of Behavioral Health
Department of Health and Social
Services
3601 C Street, Suite 934
Anchorage, AK 99503
Toll-Free: 877-266-4357 (Hotline)
Phone: 907-269-3600
Fax: 907-269-3786
Website: http://
www.hss.state.ak.us/dbh

Arizona

Division of Behavioral Health
Services
Department of Health Services
150 North 18th Avenue
Phoenix, AZ 85007
Phone: 602-542-1025
Fax: 602-542-1062
Website: http://www.azdhs.gov

Arkansas

Office of Alcohol and Drug Abuse
Prevention
Division of Behavioral Health
Services (DHHS)
4313 West Markham
Third Floor Administration
Little Rock, AR 72205
Phone: 501-686-9866
Fax: 501-686-9396
Website: http://www.arkansas.gov/
dhs/dmhs/
alco_drug_abuse_prevention.htm

California

Department of Alcohol and Drug
Programs
1700 K Street
Sacramento, CA 95811
Toll-Free: 800-879-2772
Fax: 916-323-1270
Website: http://www.adp.ca.gov
E-mail:
resourcecenter@adp.state.ca.us

Colorado

Division of Behavioral Health
Department of Human Services
3824 West Princeton Circle
Denver, CO 80236-3120
Phone: 303-866-7480
Fax: 303-866-7481
Website: http://
www.cdhs.state.co.us/adad

Connecticut

Department of Mental Health and
Addiction Services
410 Capitol Avenue, 4th Floor
P.O. Box 341431, MS #14COM
Hartford, CT 06134
Toll Free: 800-446-7348
Phone: 860-418-6962
Fax: 860-418-6690
Website: http://www.ct.gov/dmhas/
site/default.asp

Delaware

Alcohol and Drug Services
Division of Substance Abuse and
Mental Health
1901 North DuPont Highway
Administration Building, First Floor
New Castle, DE 19720
Phone: 302-255-9399
Fax: 302-255-4428
Website: http://
www.dhss.delaware.gov/dsamh/
index.html
E-mail: DHSSInfo@state.de.us

District Of Columbia

Addiction, Prevention, and
Recovery Administration
1300 First Street, N.E., Suite 300
Washington, DC 20002
Phone: 202-727-8857
Fax: 202-727-0092
Website: http://www.dchealth.dc.gov/
doh/site/default.asp

Florida

Substance Abuse Program Office
Florida Department of Children
and Families
1317 Winewood Boulevard
Building 6, Room 330
Tallahassee, FL 32399-0700
Phone: 850-487-2920
Fax: 850-487-2239
Website: http://www.dcf.state.fl.us/
mentalhealth/sa

Georgia

Addictive Diseases Program
Division of MHDDAD
2 Peachtree Street, N.W.
22nd Floor
Suite 22-273
Atlanta, GA 30303-3171
Phone: 404-657-2331
Fax: 404-657-2256
Website: http://
mhddad.dhr.georgia.gov/portal/
site/dhr-mhddad

Hawaii

Alcohol and Drug Abuse Division
Department of Health
601 Kamokila Boulevard, Room 360
Kapolei, HI 96707
Phone: 808-692-7506
Fax: 808-692-7521
Website: http://hawaii.gov/health/
substance-abuse

Idaho

Division of Behavioral Health
Department of Health and Welfare
450 West State Street, 3rd Floor
P.O. Box 83720
Boise, ID 83720-0036
Toll-Free: 800-926-2588 (Hotline)
Phone: 208-334-5935
Fax: 208-332-7305
Website: http://www.healthandwelfare
.idaho.gov/site/3460/default.aspx

Illinois

Division of Alcoholism and
Substance Abuse
Department of Human Services
100 West Randolph, Suite 5-600
Chicago, IL 60601
Phone: 312-814-3840
Fax: 312-814-2419
Website: http://www.dhs.state.il.us/
page.aspx?item=31787

Indiana

Division of Mental Health and
Addiction
Family and Social Services
Administration
402 West Washington Street
Room W353
Indianapolis, IN 46204-2739
Phone: 317-232-7800
Fax: 317-233-3472
Website: www.in.gov/fssa/dmha

Iowa

Department of Public Health
Lucas State Office Building
321 East 12th Street
Des Moines, IA 50319-0075
Phone: 515-281-4417
Fax: 515-281-4535
Website: http://
www.idph.state.ia.us/bh/
substance_abuse.asp

Kansas

SRS Health Care Policy/AAPS
DSOB 10th Floor North
915 Harrison Street
Topeka, KS 66612
Toll-Free: 800-586-3690 (Hotline)
Phone: 785-296-6807
Fax: 785-296-7275
Website: http://www.srskansas.org/
services/alc-drug_assess.htm

Kentucky

Division of Mental Health and
Substance Abuse
Department for MH/MR Services
100 Fair Oaks Lane, 4E-D
Frankfort, KY 40621
Phone: 502-564-4456
Fax: 502-564-9010
Website: http://mhmr.ky.gov/mhsas

Louisiana

Office for Addictive Disorders
Department of Health and Hospitals
628 North 4th Street, 4th Floor
P.O. Box 2790
Baton Rouge, LA 70821-2790
Phone: 225-342-6717
Fax: 225-342-3875
Website: http://www.dhh.louisiana
.gov/offices/?ID=23

Maine

Office of Substance Abuse
Department of Health and Human
Services
 41 Anthony Ave., SHS # 11
Augusta, ME 04333-0011
Phone: 207-287-2595
Fax: 207-287-4334
Website: http://www.maine.gov/
dhhs/osa
E-mail: osa.ircosa@maine.gov

Maryland

Alcohol and Drug Abuse
Administration
Department of Health and Mental
Hygiene
55 Wade Avenue
Catonsville, MD 21228
Phone: 410-402-8600
Fax: 410-402-8601
Website: http://maryland-adaa.org/
ka/index.cfm
E-mail: adaainfo@dhmh.state.md.us

Massachusetts

Bureau of Substance Abuse
Services
Department of Public Health
250 Washington Street, 3rd Floor
Boston, MA 02108-4619
Toll-Free: 800-327-5050 (Hotline)
Phone: 617-624-5111
Fax: 617-624-5185
Website: http://www.mass.gov (use
search box to locate link to Bureau)
E-mail: bsas.questions@state.ma.us

Michigan

Bureau of Substance Abuse and
Addiction Services
Office of Drug Control Policy
Department of Community Health
320 South Walnut
Lewis Cass Bldg., 5th Floor
Lansing, MI 48913
Toll-Free: 888-736-0253
Website: http://www.michigan.gov/
mdch/1,1607,7-132-2941_4871—
,00.html

Minnesota

Alcohol and Drug Abuse Division
Department of Human Services
P.O. Box 64977
Saint Paul, MN 55164-0977
Phone: 651-431-2460
Fax: 651-431-7449
Website: http://www.dhs.state.mn.us
(click on Program Contact Numbers)
E-mail: dhs.chemhealth@state.mn.us

Mississippi

Bureau of Alcohol and Drug Abuse
Department of Mental Health
1101 Robert E. Lee Building
239 North Lamar Street
Jackson, MS 39201
Phone: 601-359-1288
Fax: 601-359-6295
Website: http://www.dmh.state.ms.us/
substance_abuse.htm

Missouri

Division of Alcohol and Drug Abuse
1706 East Elm Street
P.O. Box 687
Jefferson City, MO 65102
Phone: 573-751-4942
Fax: 573-751-7814
Website: http://
www.dmh.missouri.gov/ada/
adaindex.htm
E-mail: adamail@dmh.mo.gov

Montana

Addictive and Mental Disorders
Division
Department of Public Health and
Human Services
555 Fuller
P.O. Box 202905
Helena, MT 59620-2905
Phone: 406-444-3964
Fax: 406-444-9389
Website: http://
www.dphhs.mt.gov/amdd

Nebraska

Division of Behavioral Health
Department of Health and Human
Services Systems
P.O. Box 95026
Lincoln, NE 68509-5026
Phone: 402-473-3818 (Hotline)
Phone: 402-471-7818
Fax: 402-471-7859
Website: http://www.dhhs.ne.gov/
sua/suaindex.htm
E-mail: BHDivision@dhhs.ne.gov

Nevada

Substance Abuse Prevention and
Treatment Agency
Department of Health and Human
Services
Mental Health and Development
Services
4126 Technology Way, 2nd Floor
Carson City, NV 89706
Phone: 775-684-4190
Fax: 775-684-4185
Website: http://mhds.state.nv.us

New Hampshire

Office of Alcohol and Drug Policy
Department of Health and Human
Services
105 Pleasant Street
Concord, NH 03301
Phone: 603-271-6110
Fax: 603-271-6105
Website: http://www.dhhs.state.nh.us/
dhhs/atod/a1-treatment

New Jersey

Division of Addiction Services
Department of Human Services
120 S. Stockton Street, 3rd Floor
Trenton, NJ 08611
P.O. Box 362
Trenton, NJ 08625-0362
Toll-Free: 800-238-2333 (Hotline)
Phone: 609-292-5760
Fax: 609-292-3816
Website: http://www.state.nj.us/
humanservices/das/index.htm

New Mexico

Behavioral Health Services
Division
Human Services Department
P.O. Box 2348
Santa Fe, NM 87504-1234
Toll-Free: 800-362-2013 (Hotline)
Phone: 505-476-9266
Fax: 505-476-9272
Website: http://
www.hsd.state.nm.us/bhsd

New York

New York State Office Of
Alcoholism and Substance Abuse
Services
1450 Western Avenue
Albany, NY 12203-3526
Phone: 518-473-3460
Website: http://
www.oasas.state.ny.us
E-mail:
communications@oasas.state.ny.us

North Carolina

Community Policy Management
Division of MH/DD/SA Services
325 North Salisbury St., Suite 679-C
3007 Mail Service Center
Raleigh, NC 27699-3007
Toll-Free: 800-662-7030 (Hotline)
Phone: 919-733-4670
Fax: 919-508-0962
Website: http://
www.dhhs.state.nc.us/mhddsas

North Dakota

Division of Mental Health and
Substance Abuse Services
Department of Human Services
Prairie Hills Plaza
1237 West Divide Ave., Suite 1-C
Bismarck, ND 58501
Phone: 701-328-8920
Fax: 701-328-8969
Website: http://www.nd.gov/dhs/
services/mentalhealth
E-mail: dhsmhsas@state.nd.us

Ohio

Ohio Department of Alcohol and
Drug Addiction Services
280 North High Street, 12th Floor
Columbus, OH 43215-2550
Phone: 614-752-8645 (Hotline)
Phone: 614-466-3445
Fax: 614-752-8645
Website: http://www.ada.ohio.gov
E-mail: info@ada.ohio.gov

Oklahoma

Oklahoma Department of Mental
Health and Substance Abuse
Services (ODMHSAS)
1200 N.E. 13th, Second Floor
P.O. Box 53277
Oklahoma City, OK 73152
Phone: 405-522-3908
Fax: 405-522-3650
Website: http://www.odmhsas.org

Oregon

Addictions and Mental Health
Division
Department of Human Services
500 Summer Street, N.E., E86
Salem, OR 97301-1118
Phone: 503-945-5763
Fax: 503-378-8467
Website: http://www.oregon.gov/
DHS/addiction/index.shtml
E-mail: oadap.info@state.or.us

Pennsylvania

Bureau of Drug and Alcohol
Programs
Pennsylvania Department of Health
02 Kline Plaza
Harrisburg, PA 17104
Phone: 717-783-8200
Fax: 717-783-8200
Website: http://
www.dsf.health.state.pa.us (scroll
down to Drug and Alcohol links)

Rhode Island

Division Behavioral Health and
Developmental Disabilities
Barry Hall Building
14 Harrington Road
Cranston, RI 02920
Phone: 401-462-4680
Toll-Free: 866-252-3784
Fax: 401-462-6078
Website: http://www.mhrh.ri.gov/SA

South Carolina

South Carolina Department of
Alcohol and Other Drug Abuse
Services
101 Executive Center Drive
Suite 215
Columbia, SC 29210-9498
Phone: 803-896-5555
Fax: 803-896-5557
Website: http://
www.daodas.state.sc.us

South Dakota

Division of Alcohol and Drug
Abuse
Department of Human Services
3800 East Highway 34
Hillsview Plaza
C/O 500 East Capitol
Pierre, SD 57501-5070
Phone: 605-773-3123
Fax: 605-773-7076
Website: http://dhs.sd.gov
E-mail: infodada@dhs.state.sd.us

Tennessee

Department of Mental Health and DD
Tennessee Department of Health
Cordell Hull Building, First Floor
425 Fifth Avenue North
Nashville, TN 37243
Phone: 615-741-1921
Fax: 615-532-2419
Website: http://health.state.tn.us/
index.htm

Texas

Mental Health and Substance
Abuse Division
Department of State Health Services
P. O. Box 149347
Austin, TX 78714-9347
Toll-Free: 877-966-3784 (Hotline)
Phone: 512-206-5000
Fax: 512-206-5718
Website: http://www.dshs.state.tx.us
E-mail: contact@dshs.state.tx.us

Utah

Division of Substance Abuse and
Mental Health
Utah Department of Human
Services
120 North 200 West, #209
Salt Lake City, UT 84103
Phone: 801-538-3939
Fax: 801-538-9892
Website: http://www.dsamh.utah.gov
E-mail:
dsamhwebmaster@utah.gov

Vermont

Division of Alcohol and Drug
Abuse Programs, Dept. of Health
108 Cherry Street
P.O. Box 70
Burlington, VT 05402
Phone: 802-651-1550
Fax: 802-651-1573
Website: http://healthvermont.gov
E-mail: vtadap@vdh.state.vt.us

Virginia

Office of Substance Abuse Services
Department of Mental Health,
MR, and Substance Abuse Services
P.O. Box 1797
1220 Bank Street
Richmond, VA 23218-1797
Phone: 804-786-3906
Fax: 804-786-9248
Website: http://
www.dmhmrsas.virginia.gov

Washington

Division of Alcohol and Substance
Abuse
Dept. of Social and Health Services
P.O. Box 45330
626 Eighth Ave., S.E.
Olympia, WA 98504-5330
Toll-Free: 800-562-1240 (Hotline)
Toll-Free: 877-301-4557
Fax: 360-586-0341
Website: http://www1.dshs.wa.gov/
DASA
E-mail: DASA@dshs.wa.gov

West Virginia

Division on Alcoholism and Drug
Abuse
Office of Behavioral Health Services
Department of Health and Human
Resources
350 Capitol Street, Room 350
Charleston, WV 25301-3702
Phone: 304-558-0627
Fax: 304-558-1008
Website: http://www.wvdhhr.org/
bhhf/ada.asp
E-mail: obhs@wvdhhr.org

Wisconsin

Bureau of Mental Health and
Substance Abuse Services
1 West Wilson Street, Room 850
P.O. Box 7851
Madison, WI 53707-7851
Phone: 608-266-2717
Fax: 608-266-1533
Website: http://dhs.wisconsin.gov/
substabuse/index.htm

Wyoming

Substance Abuse Division
Department of Health
6101 Yellowstone Road, Suite 220
Cheyenne, WY 82002-0480
Toll-Free: 800-535-4006
Phone: 307-777-6494
Fax: 307-777-5849
Website: http://wdh.state.wy.us/
mhsa/index.html

Index

Index

Page numbers that appear in *Italics* refer to illustrations. Page numbers that have a small 'n' after the page number refer to information shown as Notes at the beginning of each chapter. Page numbers that appear in **Bold** refer to information contained in boxes on that page (except Notes information at the beginning of each chapter).